WORLD BANK WORKING PAPER NO. 20

W9-AXK-620

HIV/AIDS and Tuberculosis in Central Asia

Country Profiles

Joana Godinho
Thomas Novotny
Hiwote Tadesse
Anatoly Vinokur

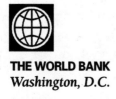

THE WORLD BANK
Washington, D.C.

ISBN: 0-8213-5687-9
eISBN: 0-8213-5688-7
ISSN: 1726-5878

Joana Godinho is Senior Health Specialist in the Human Development Department, and Hiwote Tadesse is a Program Assistant in the Environment and Sustainable Development Department, Europe and Central Asia Region, The World Bank. Thomas Novotny is the Director of International Programs at the University of California, San Francisco, and Anatoly Vinokur is the Health Deputy Programme Manager Health for DFID in Russia.

Library of Congress Cataloging-in-Publication Data has been requested.

TABLE OF CONTENTS

TABLES

FIGURES

ABSTRACT

The countries of Central Asia are still at the earliest stages of an HIV/AIDS epidemic. However, there is cause for serious concern due to: the steep growth of new HIV cases in the region; the established related epidemics of injecting drug use, sexually transmitted infections (STIs) and tuberculosis (TB); youth representing more than 40 percent of the total regional population; and the low levels of knowledge about the epidemics. The underlying causes for the interlinked epidemics of drug abuse, HIV/AIDS, STIs and TB in Central Asia are many, including drug production in Afghanistan and its distribution throughout the Former Soviet Union (FSU); unemployment among youth; imprisonment for drug use; overcrowding in prisons; and striking levels of poverty.

HIV/AIDS and tuberculosis may have a potentially devastating effect on human capital, economic development, and health systems reform. In Russia, economic analysis has described the significant future impact on health and health systems if the concentrated epidemic in that country goes unchecked (Ruhl etal. 2002). The opportunity for prevention in low prevalence environments provides an imperative for action, because when HIV prevalence among high-risk groups reaches 20 percent or more, prevention is no longer possible and expensive treatment for AIDS and related opportunistic infections will overwhelm under funded health care systems such as those in Central Asia. Low prevalence, or nascent epidemics of HIV create little incentive for focused attention. However, through careful consideration of the potential for these epidemics to grow, the World Bank can help client countries incorporate effective prevention strategies into health systems development projects or into specific public health projects to address these infections.

Therefore, to address this impending crisis, the World Bank has initiated the study of HIV/AIDS, STIs, and TB in Central Asia. The Central Asia HIV/AIDS and TB Country Profiles were developed to inform Bank management and other stakeholders about the main characteristics of the epidemics in the sub region; to describe differences among the countries; and to develop an understanding of the main issues related to the prevention of HIV/AIDS and the control of TB. The Country Profiles summarize information available from Governments and partner organizations such as the UN agencies, USAID, and the Soros Foundation/OSI. It covers the following aspects: epidemiology; strategic and regulatory frameworks; surveillance; preventive, diagnostic, and treatment activities; non-governmental (NGO) and partner activities; and funding resources available. The Country Profiles are based on review of existing statistics and reports and on discussions with key stakeholders – Governments, donors, and NGOs – during several missions to Central Asia. In the following pages, we summarize the main issues identified in the initial assessment and the main recommendations for further study and action.

Further studies focusing on HIV/AIDS are being prepared for publication, with the following objectives:

(i) Estimate the potential epidemiological and economic impact of the HIV/AIDS epidemic in Central Asia;
(ii) Identify key stakeholders and their roles in controlling the epidemic;
(iii) Identify gaps in strategies, policies and legislation aimed at controlling the epidemic;
(iv) Assess the institutional capacity, including of public health services and NGOs, to control the epidemic; and
(v) Prepare the Bank's communication strategy on HIV/AIDS in Central Asia.

The Bank has initiated a Central Asia TB Study. It has also initiated the preparation of HIV/AIDS Components of Health Projects in Tajikistan and Uzbekistan, and is considering the possibility of assisting regional Governments in preparing a Central Asia HIV/AIDS and TB Project. Such a project would include regional and country-specific components, and would be partly financed by IDA grants.

ACKNOWLEDGMENTS

This report was written by Joana Godinho, who manages the Central Asia AIDS and TB Studies, based on the draft report from co-authors and existing reports from regional Governments and partner institutions. Hiwote Tadesse and Anatoly Vinokur collected the data and wrote the first drafts, respectively, of the HIV/AIDS and TB Country Profiles. Natalya Beisenova, Dinara Djoldosheva, Jamshed Khasanov, Saodat Bazarova, Guljahan Kurbanova, and Dilnara Isamiddinova provided data and organized meetings with counterparts and other stakeholders in their respective countries: Kazakhstan, Kyrgyz Republic, Tajikistan, Turkmenistan, and Uzbekistan. Thomas Novotny revised and Linda Currie edited these Country Profiles; Gizella Diaz prepared for publication.

The Central Asia AIDS Study Peer Reviewers were Martha Ainsworth, Diana Weil, Karl Dehne, and Nina Schwalbe, but many others have provided insightful comments.

The study team is grateful to the Ministries of Health, Justice, and Internal Affairs; AIDS Centers and TB Institutes from Central Asian countries; and all regional partners and NGOs that provided data and participated in meetings to discuss the main issues identified.

The World Bank

Vice President:	Shigeo Katsu
Country Director:	Dennis de Tray
Sector Director:	Michal Rutkowski
Sector Manager:	Armin Fidler
Task Team Leader:	Joana Godinho

ACRONYMS

AIDS	Acquired Immune Deficiency Syndrome
CAR	Central Asia Republics
CCM	Country Coordination Mechanism
CDC	Center for Disease Control and Prevention
CSW	Commercial Sex Worker
DFID	Department for International Development
DOTS	TB Directly Observed Therapy Short-Course
ECA	Europe and Central Asia
ESCM	Electronic Surveillance Case-Based Management System
FSU	Former Soviet Union
FPG	Family Practice Group
GDF	Global Drug Fund
GFATM	Global Fund to Fight AIDS, TB & Malaria
HFA	Health for All
HIV	Human Immunodeficiency Virus
HR	Harm Reduction
IDA	International Development Association
IDU	Intravenous Drug Use
IEC	Information, Education and Communication Campaign
IFRC	International Federation of Red Cross
IHRD	International Harm Reduction Development
IHRP	International Harm Reduction Program
IOM	International Organization for Migration
IPPF	International Planned Parenthood Federation
IUATLD	International Union against Tuberculosis and Lung Disease
KAP	Knowledge, Attitudes and Practices
KfW	German Development Bank (Kreditanstalt für Wiederaufbau)
MDGs	Millennium Development Goals
MDRTB	Multi-Drug Resistant Tuberculosis
MMR	Mass Miniature Radiography (fluorography)
MOH	Ministry of Health
MOIA	Ministry of Internal Affaires
MOJ	Ministry of Justice
MSF	Médecins Sans Frontières
MSM	Men who have sex with men
MTCT	Mother to Child Transmission
NGO	Non Governmental Organization
NTP	National Tuberculosis Program
OECD	Organization for Economic Cooperation and Development
PLWHA	People Living with HIV/AIDS
PRM	Participatory Resource Mapping
PSI	Population Services International
RAR	Rapid Assessment Response
STI	Sexually Transmitted Infection
TB	Tuberculosis
TG	UN AIDS Thematic Group
TOR	Terms of Reference
UNAIDS	Joint United Nations Program on HIV/AIDS

UNDP	United Nations Development Program
UNFPA	United Nations Fund for Population Assistance
UNHCR	UN High Commission on Refugees
UNICEF	United Nations International Children's Fund
UNODCCP	UN Office for Drug Control and Crime Prevention
USAID	United States Agency for International Development
VCT	Voluntary testing and counseling
VDRL	Venereal Disease Research Laboratory (test for syphilis)
WHO	World Health Organization

MAIN ISSUES

Extent and Likely Impact of the HIV/AIDS Epidemic in Central Asia

The HIV/AIDS epidemic is still at a low level in the countries of Central Asia, but this situation presents a dual challenge: first, to call attention to the projected epidemic so that policy-makers at the national level understand what lies ahead, given international evidence on the growth of HIV infection; and second, to plan, in the context of extremely limited resources, a rational response to HIV/AIDS throughout the sub region. In Central Asia, as in the rest of ECA, the epidemic is rather significantly under-measured, but it is clear to all that HIV incidence is increasing, following epidemics of intravenous drug use (IDU) and sexually transmitted illnesses (STI) throughout these countries. According Euro-HIV, countries in Central Asia have shown dramatic increases in numbers and rates of infection between 1996 and 2001 (Table 1).

Some of these increases are due to improved surveillance of HIV infection (this phenomenon is known as *reporting artifact*), but nevertheless, all data point to a rapidly increasing epidemic. Official prevalence estimates of HIV infection among the adult populations vary between 0.14 percent in Kazakhstan to less than 0.01 percent in Tajikistan, Turkmenistan, and Uzbekistan (Table 2).

All Governments agree that drug trafficking and intravenous drug use have increased since 1995, most dramatically since the 2001 war in Afghanistan. When frontiers in Tajikistan and Uzbekistan opened, the prices of drugs decreased. Although the majority (60–90 percent) of reported HIV cases is among intravenous drug users, the proportion of cases attributed to heterosexual transmission has also been growing recently. Globally, IDUs, commercial sex workers (CSWs), men who have sex with men (MSM), and young people in general are recognized as the groups most at risk of HIV/AIDS. The overlap between IDUs and CSWs in this sub region is considered an added risk for transmission of the epidemic from highly vulnerable groups to vulnerable groups such as young people. Furthermore, occasional CSW practiced by female students and underreported homosexual behavior may present additional risks for rapid spread of the epidemic to youth in general. School dropouts, who are especially at risk of IDU and CSW, may deserve more targeted attention than they receive at present. Mobile populations such as truck drivers,

TABLE 1. RATE OF GROWTH OF HIV EPIDEMIC IN CENTRAL ASIA

Country	1996		2001		
	Cases	Rate per million	Cases	Rate per million	Cumulative total
Kazakhstan	48	2.9	1,175	72.6	2,522
Kyrgyz Rep.	2	0.4	149	31.5	202
Tajikistan	0	0	34	5.4	45
Uzbekistan	0	0	549	22.2	779

Source: Hamers FF and Downs AM. HIV in Central and Eastern Europe. *Lancet* February 28, 2003.

mariners, the homeless, refugees, migrant workers, and trafficked women are also among the highly vulnerable groups, including in neighboring countries such as China. Therefore, it is expected that the incidence of HIV will increase among them in Central Asia as well. Trafficking of drugs, and women and children for prostitution, is of particular concern. Prisoners and institutionalized children are other groups that deserve additional study and targeted programs.

Officially reported cumulative HIV cases are shown in Table 3. However, Centers for Disease Control and Prevention (CDC) surveillance data in Central Asia indicate that the total number of people living with HIV/AIDS is estimated to be about 90,000. Based upon projections for the year 2005, this number will rise to 1.65 million without concerted efforts to target interventions.[1] This growth may create a catastrophic impact at the household level and a significant impact on health services expenditures at the national level.

The Public Health Approach in Central Asia: Early Efforts

The Governments of Kazakhstan, Kyrgyz Republic, Tajikistan and Uzbekistan have approved HIV/AIDS Strategies prepared with assistance from the Joint United Nations Program on HIV/AIDS (UNAIDS).[2] These countries have established high-level multi-sectoral committees to coordinate strategy implementation. The situation is more tenuous in Turkmenistan, but the UNAIDS Thematic Group (TG) is assisting the Government to prepare a Strategy. The Strategies include multi-sectoral approaches and evidence-based interventions to the epidemic (Ball 1998,

TABLE 2. THE HIV/AIDS EPIDEMIC IN CENTRAL ASIA

	Year HIV first reported	# People living w/ HIV/AIDS	Prevalence (adults)	Predominant mode of transmission
Kazakhstan	1989	3,448	0.14	IDU
Kyrgyz R.	1987	410	0.01	IDU
Tajikistan	1991	92	<0.01	IDU
Turkmenistan	1997	1	<0.01	Nosocomial
Uzbekistan	1992	2,209	<0.01	IDU
Central Asia	1987–92	5,904	<0.01	IDU

Source: national statistics (March 2003 Kazakhstan; May 2003 Kyrgyz Republic; April 2003 Tajikistan and Uzbekistan).

---

1. http://www.usaid.gov/regions/europe_eurasia/car/briefers/hivaids_prevention.html. March 2003.
2. UNAIDS (2001). UNAIDS Assisted Response to HIV/AIDS, STIs and Drug Abuse in Central Asian countries. Almaty: UNAIDS – Central Asia.

TABLE 3. NEWLY-DIAGNOSED HIV INFECTIONS IN CENTRAL ASIA								
	Up to 1995	1996	1997	1998	1999	2000	2001	2002	Total
Kazakhstan	31	48	437	299	185	347	1,175	735	3,257
Kyrgyz Republic	17	2	2	6	10	16	149	160	362
Tajikistan	2	0	1	1	0	7	34	30	75
Turkmenistan	–	–	–	–	–	–	2	–	2
Uzbekistan	38	–	7	3	28	154	780	2,000	3,010
Central Asia	88	50	447	309	223	524	2,140	2,925	6,706

Source: European Center on AIDS Monitoring, Central Asia Ministries of Health (Total refers to December 2002 for Kazakhstan; May 2003 for the Kyrgyz Republic; April 2003 for Tajikistan; and June 2002 for Uzbekistan).

Burrows 2001): establishment of sentinel surveillance, harm reduction (HR),[3] prevention and treatment of STIs, and education of young people in general. All countries have approved AIDS-related laws, are implementing multi-year and multi-sectoral programs to prevent further spread of HIV/AIDS, and have functional UNAIDS TGs, with Government, partner organizations, and NGO representation. However, strategy implementation is still quite limited throughout the sub region due to lack of political leadership, inadequate public knowledge, and limited funding for prevention.

Issues surrounding the legal framework on the production, sale, and use of drugs to treat HIV and related diseases; CSWs; homosexuality; and prevention and treatment of STIs varies from country to country. It is more advanced in Kazakhstan and Kyrgyz Republic and more conservative in Uzbekistan and Turkmenistan. The Government of Kazakhstan is considering decriminalization of drug use. The Kyrgyz Republic Parliament is reviewing a new Drug Law that softens penalties for drug use and could eventually consider decriminalization. Decriminalization of drug use is highly controversial, but Organization for Economic Cooperation and Development (OECD) countries such as Netherlands, Switzerland, and Portugal have adopted this approach (Van Het Loo etal. 2001; Swiss Expert Commission 1996). Decriminalization may facilitate HIV/AIDS prevention efforts through destigmatization of IDUs, and it would diminish overcrowding in prisons, thereby reducing detention costs and TB transmission. Potential savings could be used to buy supplies (condoms, syringes) necessary for prevention of HIV/AIDS and pharmaceuticals necessary to treat TB, HIV/AIDS, and STIs.

Governments, UN agencies, bilateral agencies, and national and international NGOs are involved in prevention activities such as harm reduction and school-based reproductive health education throughout Central Asia, but these occur only as pilot activities. Scaling up prevention activities to cover the groups at most risk is needed to impact the epidemic, but Governments do not have the political will or resources necessary to do so. UN agencies have funded initial work with highly vulnerable groups, and most HR programs are implemented by the Soros Foundation/OSI through NGOS in Central Asian countries.

Additional resources and capacity will be necessary to: provide groups at risk with voluntary anonymous testing, education, and counseling (VCT); promote/market safer sex; treat STIs; provide replacement therapy for IDU; reduce demand for drugs; build capacity of public health services and NGOs to tackle the epidemic; and increase the political will and public knowledge necessary to address the epidemic openly and effectively. Former drug users and CSWs can be

---

3. Harm reduction is the name given to outreach programs that include peer education, counseling and testing, needle exchange, and provision of condoms to highly vulnerable groups. It has proven to be very cost-effective in developing and developed countries. (See, for example, Commonwealth of Australia 2002. Return on Investment in Needle and Syringe Programs in Australia.)

trained to engage in peer education about harm reduction and safe sex. More information is needed to determine the optimum approach to Mother to Child Transmission (MTCT) in the sub region. Currently, there are few data on the extent of this mode of transmission, while costs for screening all pregnant women may be quite excessive and not cost-effective in the current low-level epidemic situation.

Public Advocacy and Education

Evidence about knowledge, attitudes, and practices among decision-makers, opinion-makers, and health professionals about HIV/AIDS is deficient in the sub region. Some stakeholders (Governments, donors, and NGOs) are well aware of the IDU epidemic and the resulting growth of the HIV epidemic. However, all stakeholders recognize the low level of knowledge among health professionals, the low level of awareness about HIV/AIDS among highly vulnerable groups, and the low level of knowledge about the disease, and high level of stigmatization of people living with HIV/AIDS (PLWHA) among the general population. While some Government counterparts (Kazakhstan, Kyrgyz Republic, Tajikistan) are aware of the need to take action on politically difficult measures, others (Uzbekistan, Turkmenistan) are reluctant to address issues such as decriminalization of drug use, HR, and replacement therapy (for example, with non-injectable drugs such as methadone). School education on preventing IDU, STIs, and HIV/AIDS is still very limited, although United Nations International Children's Fund (UNICEF) is investing significant resources to scale up this program throughout Central Asia (UNICEF 2002).

Many NGOs are active in programs to prevent HIV/AIDS throughout the region, funded by international organizations such as the Soros Foundation/OSI. However, the lack of inter-ministerial cooperation, poor NGO and donor coordination, and poor NGO-donor-Government coordination may pose significant obstacles to effective HIV/AIDS control strategies. In particular, controversial strategies, even though based on solid scientific evidence, are affected by bilateral donor political influences. Public health services and NGOs occasionally cooperate, but partnerships, which may include transfer of funds from the public sector to the NGO sector, should be better developed to ensure coverage of high-risk groups. Integrating NGOs through periodic roundtables and Government funding have been suggested as remedies.

With the exception of Turkmenistan, all Central Asian Governments are developing a regional partnership to decrease IDU and to confront the IDU-based epidemic of HIV/AIDS (see statement from Regional Conference on Drug Abuse in Central Asia, in June, in Taskhent[4]).

Funding of HIV/AIDS and STI Programs

Most FSU governments are not able to report on expenditures to address HIV/AIDS and STIs. This is partly due to the fact that line item budgets cover inputs such as human resources and pharmaceuticals but not whole programs, and partly due to the secrecy that still dominates some FSU countries. Nevertheless, it is clear that funding available from the public budgets to prevent and treat HIV/AIDS is very limited in all countries.

Because of the renewed focus on poverty through the Millennium Development Goals (MDGs) and because of the war in Afghanistan, Central Asia has become a focus of international political attention. Several organizations have been providing financial and/or technical assistance for research and intervention on HIV/AIDS, STIs, and TB; these include UN agencies, bilateral agencies such as USAID, the German Development Bank (KfW) and Department for International Development (DFID), and international NGOs such as the Soros Foundation/OSI, and the AIDS Foundation East West. These partnerships need continued development and funding. However,

---

4. Regional Conference on Drug Abuse in Central Asia. Situation Assessment and Responses. Tashkent: UNODCCP, WHO, USAID, OSCE, Austrian Federal Ministry of Foreign Affairs and Government of Uzbekistan.

available indigenous capacity only allows for limited research and pilot activities but not scaling up of these activities to cover high-risk groups and marginalized populations, let alone the bridge populations to other groups.

More than $15 million is immediately necessary to cover the estimated number of IDUs in Central Asia using a package of services including disposable syringes, condoms, and education about the transmission of the infection. However, given the large numbers and inaccessibility of IDUs, this figure might be a gross underestimation of needs, especially with respect to the supply of needles and the resources necessary to distribute them. Pilot programs reach only a few thousand IDUs, and thus scaling up will require enormous additional resources. According to recent estimates, about US$ 1 billion would be necessary for HIV/AIDS prevention and treatment in Central Asia in the period 2004–2007 (Futures Group and Instituto Nacional de Salud Publica 2003).

The Global Fund to Fight AIDS, Tuberculosis and Malaria (GFATM) may provide a significant source of funding to the sub region. Kazakhstan, Kyrgyz Republic, Tajikistan and Uzbekistan have already been awarded grants from the GFATM for HIV/AIDS for 2003–2004, and the International Development Association (IDA) may award additional grants to Kyrgyz, Tajikistan and Uzbekistan in the near future.

There is the risk, however, that if significant funding becomes available in the near future, Governments might consider that prevention activities are covered by international organizations, and allocate Government funds mainly to diagnosis and treatment activities. As the funding available from other sources is not enough to cover all necessary prevention activities, further spread of the epidemic will not be prevented. Furthermore, there is the risk that inappropriate treatment with anti-retroviral drugs will create resistance, as it has been observed throughout the region with inappropriate use of TB drugs. This would complicate significantly the public health approach to HIV/AIDS in the sub region. It might be appropriate, in fact, to limit anti-retroviral treatment schemes to pilots to assure that such regimens can be implemented, including laboratory monitoring, procurement, patient compliance, and health care quality assurance.

Extent of the Tuberculosis Epidemic

The TB situation in Central Asian countries generally fits the pattern of the TB epidemic in Eastern Europe in the 1990s. Kazakhstan bears the largest burden of TB in the region, with almost 50,000 cases of active TB registered in 2001. About 25,000 new cases of TB and 5,000 deaths were reported each year in the late 1990s. The specific number of cases in each country is debatable because case notification is incomplete. For example, in Tajikistan only 10 percent of the estimated smear-positive sputum cases were reported in 2000. Prison data are only variably included in the national TB statistics in these countries as well. Nonetheless, Central Asia has reported the highest TB death rates in the FSU. In the latter 1990s, reported TB incidence rates in Kazakhstan and Kyrgyz Republic even surpassed those in the Russian Federation. Although there is no systematic surveillance of multi-drug resistant TB (MDRTB), rates of MDRTB in some areas of Central Asia and in prisons are believed to be amongst the highest in the world. Serious concerns remain about TB in the sub region: (i) there is an unwillingness or lack of ability of Governments to allocate the necessary funding for DOTS implementation at the national level, including in prisons; (ii) there is inefficiency in utilization of available public resources and donor funding; and (iii) the treatment of MDRTB in Kazakhstan and Kyrgyz Republic before satisfactory DOTS implementation is ill advised.

TB surveillance varies across the Central Asian countries. In Kazakhstan, the TB Electronic Surveillance Case-Based Management System (ESCM), developed with assistance of the US CDC, became fully operational throughout the country in 2000, but it is unclear whether it is still in use; in Kyrgyz Republic, surveillance is case-based reporting according to World Health Organization (WHO) standards; in other countries surveillance is mostly carried out according to the old Soviet reporting system, or in pilot Directly Observed Treatment Short-Course (DOTS) programs by WHO and international NGOs such as Medecins Sans Frontieres (MSF) and Project HOPE. Consequently, case notification rates vary considerably across the sub region (Table 4).

TABLE 4. TB CASE NOTIFICATION RATES IN CENTRAL ASIA (Estimated percentage of smear-positive cases reported)					
	1996	**1997**	**1998**	**1999**	**2000**
Kazakhstan	73.6	55.1	78.8	73.4	80.0
Kyrgyz Rep.	72.4	77.0	41.4	60.1	38.0
Tajikistan	6.5	15.9	18.3	NA	10.0
Turkmenistan	41.4	54.1	55.0	54.0	56.0
Uzbekistan	58.3	40.1	40.8	38.0	33.0
CAR					47.0
FSU					36.0
Central Europe					51.0
Western Europe					36.0
Total Europe					39.0

Source: Global TB Control, WHO reports 1998–2002

The TB problem is notable with respect to the HIV/AIDS epidemic. TB in many regions of the world is the chief opportunistic infection causing mortality among HIV/AIDS patients. Thus, control of TB is interrelated with HIV prevention, particularly in closed environments such as prisons, where confined space leads to increased TB risk, and deprivation leads to IV drug use as well as homosexual risk behavior. TB in prisons is known to be an epidemiological pump that fuels generalized epidemics in other parts of the ECA region. Little has been done as yet to address HIV within prisons populations, but as both TB and HIV tend to co-exist in such closed environments, it is likely that dual epidemics will be observed among prison populations. Given the relatively large burdens of TB described above, it is also likely that there will be overlap of these epidemics in the general population unless effective prevention methods are implemented. In particular, special attention is needed to assure that TB-infected and partially treated prisoners are followed through public health and social service mechanisms to assure completion of TB therapy. In addition, it is also likely that VCT for all TB patients will be en effective prevention approach for HIV in this population.

DOTS Implementation

All countries have adopted the WHO-recommended DOTS approach. However, there are several concerns regarding TB treatment in the region: (i) there is limited coverage and implementation of DOTS, as reflected in the low treatment success rates and high rates of MDRTB; (ii) there is also partial or total lack of coverage within prisons, which are considered the epidemiological pump for the TB epidemic in the region; and (iii) in some countries, TB specialists tend to start treatment with second-line drugs before satisfactory DOTS implementation.

DOTS coverage varies significantly across the region, from Kyrgyz Republic and Kazakhstan with almost 100 percent of the population covered with DOTS, to Turkmenistan with 34 percent population coverage, to Uzbekistan with quite slow DOTS implementation, and lastly to Tajikistan, where DOTS program was halted because of civil war (Table 5). TB treatment success is only moderate in those Central Asian countries that have implemented DOTS. Kyrgyz Republic, where DOTS was first introduced in the region, ranks the best, but the treatment success rate was still below the WHO target of 85 percent cure rates in patients newly registered for treatment in 1999 (Table 6). The role of drug resistance and HIV infection needs to be investigated for better understanding of TB control efforts in the region. Central Asian countries are not yet prepared for the potential overlap between the HIV/AIDS and TB epidemics. TB is the main opportunistic disease of AIDS. Projections carried out in Russia have shown that, even in the presence of only a moderate HIV/AIDS epidemic, TB may become uncontrollable (Vinokur etal. 2001). The vertical TB

TABLE 5. POPULATION COVERAGE WITH DOTS (%)					
	1996	1997	1998	1999	2000
Kazakhstan	No DOTS	No DOTS	4	100	100
Kyrgyz	5.3	5	100	100	100
Tajikistan	No DOTS	No DOTS	0	3	0
Turkmenistan	No DOTS	No DOTS	0	0	34
Uzbekistan	No DOTS	No DOTS	2	2	7

Source: Global TB control, WHO reports 1998–2002

and HIV/AIDS approaches in Central Asia are not yet integrated, and there is lack of clarity about responsibilities for treatment of AIDS patients with TB.

Kazakhstan and Kyrgyz Republic have asked the GFATM for funds to scale up DOTS Plus, which is an extension of the time used for DOTS treatment and use of second-line drugs for treatment. However, this may be premature, given that DOTS has not been fully implemented and that there is no systematic surveillance of MDRTB. In addition, the treatment protocols used in many of the FSU countries are not evidence-based. There is, therefore, a risk of establishing resistance to second-line drugs, as with first-line drugs, due to inappropriate usage, leaving the region and the world at large with an additional public health dilemma.

Funding of TB Programs

Reported allocations for TB Programs vary from $32 million in Kazakhstan ($640/patient), in 2001, to $1.3 million in Kyrgyz Republic ($100/patient) in 2000, while data are not available for the other countries. Kazakhstan, Kyrgyz Republic, and Tajikistan have obtained funding from the GFATM. The grant plans include scaling up DOTS and, in the Kazakhstan and Kyrgyz Republic, piloting or scaling up treatment of MDRTB with second-line drugs.

NGO and Partner Activity

Several international NGOs and organizations have been assisting the Governments of Central Asia to adopt and implement the DOTS Strategy, and they have also had a key role in surveillance, diagnosis, and treatment of TB in the region. WHO provides technical assistance for DOTS implementation throughout Central Asia. USAID/CAR, through Project HOPE and CDC, has been assisting DOTS pilot projects in all Central Asian countries, including in prisons. This assistance includes upgrading surveillance systems and laboratories and training TB specialists and other health professionals on proper diagnosis and treatment of TB. MSF has supported DOTS pilot projects in the Aral Sea region in Turkmenistan and Uzbekistan, where TB rates are especially high. KfW, the German Development Bank, has been providing grants for procurement of first-line drugs, laboratory equipment, and supplies in Kyrgyz Republic and Uzbekistan. The Global

TABLE 6. TREATMENT SUCCESS					
	1995	1996	1997	1998	1999
Kazakhstan	NA	NA	74.3	79.0	79.0
Kyrgyz	NA	87.5	75.6	82.0	83.0
Tajikistan	87.6	81.8	74.5	NA	NA
Turkmenistan	73.2	63.7	58.9	NA	60.0
Uzbekistan	78.1	NA	NA	78.0	79.0

Source: Global TB control, WHO reports 1998–2002

Drug Facility has also provided first line drugs to Tajikistan. The International Federation of the Red Cross provides food and other supplies for TB patients.

The World Bank has also provided financial and technical support for DOTS implementation in Kazakhstan, Kyrgyz Republic, and Uzbekistan through health projects that have been implemented in those countries. In Kazakhstan, the Bank-financed project has closed, but the Government and the Bank are co-financing sector work, which involves a review of the TB Program. In Kyrgyz Republic, the Bank-financed project is under implementation, and additional sector work may also be eventually carried out in this area. In Uzbekistan, the Health I project is under implementation, and the Government is preparing with Bank assistance the Health II Project, which may continue to support scaling up the DOTS implementation throughout the country.

Health System Issues in Central Asia

Initial estimates of actual and projected cases of HIV and AIDS are based on incomplete and unreliable information. Three sources of data are used in the Country Profiles: official statistics (passively collected in most cases); Government and NGO estimates of IDUs and other groups at risk; and occasional sentinel surveillance data (special studies). Official data provided by the Ministries of Health cover required reported HIV/AIDS cases as well as IDUs under treatment and estimated CSWs. However, UNAIDS has estimated the number of IDUs and HIV-positive cases to exceed registered cases by 5- to 10-fold. Although Ministries of Health, partner organizations, and NGOs have carried out several seroprevalence and behavioral studies, evidence for actual seroprevalence as well as knowledge, attitudes, and practices (KAP) among groups most at risk and youth in general is still scant. Using US Agency for International Development (USAID) resources, CDC is initiating sentinel seroprevalence and behavioral surveys in Kazakhstan and Uzbekistan, and it is providing technical assistance and equipment necessary to establish sentinel surveillance throughout the region for the highly vulnerable groups (USAID/CAR 2002).

One of the major issues involving both HIV/AIDS and TB is the way in which specific illnesses are compartmentalized within FSU health systems. For example, HIV is tested and AIDS treated generally only in a referral infectious disease setting; TB may be separately managed in a pulmonary or TB hospital; prison systems have a separate hospital system; and IDU is treated in narcology centers, if at all. There is a lack of an overriding public health approach that integrates information systems, monitoring and evaluation of risks, communications, and social services. In many cases, the World Bank may support this lack of integration through health systems development projects that manifest as independent segments. These problems require an integrated approach, working across sectors, with a sense of common purpose. There is a lack of integration and cooperation among primary health care and specialized hospital services, specialized AIDS Centers, TB Institutes and Dispensaries, and the Dermatology and Venereal Disease Institutes for prevention and treatment of STIs, HIV/AIDS, and opportunistic infections, of which TB is the main one. STI syndromic case management needs to be better developed, both to reduce morbidity and to reduce the risk of HIV transmission through ulcerative STIs. Hospitals, TB services, and oncological dispensaries are expected to provide treatment of AIDS opportunistic diseases as well as palliative care, but this depends on correct diagnosis, appropriate referral, and availability of anti-retroviral drugs and monitoring systems to support their use. Anti-retroviral treatment of HIV/AIDS is not yet available throughout the region due to its high cost. For example, in Kazakhstan, only children under 15 and infected pregnant women have access to anti-retroviral treatment. If the epidemic grows as expected, both the demand for such treatment and the infrastructure necessary to support it will drain health resources from other important priorities. (These include the growing epidemic of cardiovascular and neoplastic diseases throughout the sub region, diseases which also require significant tertiary medical resources.)

Health systems in general are under-financed in the sub region. This under-financing will create a future tragedy of large proportions if prevention activities, as outlined below, are not addressed and scaled up. Even if sufficient funding is available, there may not be enough local capacity (public services and NGOs) to scale up activities for the majority of groups at risk. Throughout the region, recently established AIDS treatment and support services are still considered relatively unimportant, which raises issues of lack of power among the vulnerable groups to assert needs and lack of institutional capacity to integrate services. In addition, institutional barriers, such as the tradition of dermatology and venerealogical services should be addressed in the implementation of effective and integrated HIV/AIDS and STIs strategies. Building local institutional capacity, which is necessary in order to integrate HIV/AIDS into existing structures, was identified as one of the most urgent tasks in Tajikistan, Turkmenistan, and Uzbekistan.

Health systems in Central Asia have suffered deterioration with respect to disease surveillance as well as coverage for treatment of infectious diseases. This deterioration is an important determinant of success of prevention activities because treatment of STIs, particularly ulcerative diseases such as syphilis and chancroid, is essential to preventing spread of HIV. Moreover, functional STI treatment systems, coupled with voluntary counseling and testing of all patients for HIV, is an important component of prevention (Bos etal. 2002). The risks for HIV spread are identical to those for other STIs.

Additional financing issues revolve around underserved and thus highly vulnerable populations. Migrants, mobile populations, CSWs, and other hard-to-reach groups often do not have rights to health care, either because of registration status, social isolation, or because of inhospitable health care facilities. In addition, corruption within health care systems, may force vulnerable populations to pay out-of-pocket expenses in the form of bribes or 'envelope' money before services are rendered. Youth-friendly clinics are not as yet a commonly accepted method of reaching at-risk youth. Thus, highly vulnerable populations may not be appropriately treated, either for STIs, TB or HIV-related complications. TB and HIV demand careful follow-up, and if patients with these infections cannot or will not access services, drug resistance will develop (to both TB drugs and antiretrovirals), thus complicating the control of these infectious diseases at the global level. To address this issue, financing options that support the control of infectious diseases as a public good are needed. It is not enough to simply implement a health insurance system, but rather a public goods system of financing critical medications for global public health problems is needed. The World Bank needs to confront this need in its work on health financing systems. Privatization in the context of communicable diseases control has limited utility, and insufficient financing of pharmaceutical systems in this context provides a significant barrier to control HIV/AIDS and TB.

RECOMMENDATIONS

Recommendations for Immediate Action

For Regional Governments

1) **Improvements in Surveillance.** Regional Governments, with assistance from USAID/CAR and CDC, should scale up or initiate efforts to establish sentinel surveillance[5] of HIV/AIDS, and to improve surveillance of STIs, TB, MDRTB and DOTS implementation. Furthermore, it is essential to know more about the prevalence of risk behaviors among IDU and CSW, transfusions with unscreened blood in the sub region, and prevalence of HIV among highly vulnerable groups such as CSWs, trafficked women, migrants, truckers, and other target populations. Only through the improvement of surveillance systems can effective interventions be planned and evaluated and to know with more certainty the growth rate or control of the HIV/AIDS epidemic.

2) **Adoption and Implementation of HIV/AIDS, STIs, and TB Strategies.** The Governments of Kazakhstan, Kyrgyz Republic, Tajikistan and Uzbekistan should scale up the implementation of the approved HIV/AIDS strategies to ensure that the spread of HIV is contained, and all Governments should identify and allocate sufficient funding for DOTS implementation. The Government of Turkmenistan should approve as soon as possible a HIV/AIDS Strategies prepared with assistance from UNAIDS.

3) **Scaling Up Work with Highly Vulnerable and Vulnerable Groups.** It is necessary to quickly scale up the HIV/AIDS prevention efforts targeted at highly vulnerable groups such as IDUs, CSWs, MSM, and young people, especially unemployed or institutionalized young people. Governments should resist the temptation to invest in mass testing of the

---

5. Sentinel surveillance allows monitoring of the population's epidemic through small-scale sampling of specific subgroups. It can include special studies of HIV prevalence in highly vulnerable populations such as IDUs, anonymous and unlinked testing of blood obtained for other purposes such as in blood donations, and testing of institutionalized or military populations on a regular basis.

general population (which will have low cost-benefit and may in fact be stigmatizing to some) and comprehensive treatment with anti-retrovirals before treatment protocols, monitoring systems, and adequate prevention efforts are better implemented.

4) **Satisfactory Implementation of the DOTS Strategy.** All Governments should focus on scaling up DOTS implementation throughout their countries, including prisons, and obtaining satisfactory results. The Governments of Kazakhstan and Kyrgyz should postpone use of TB second-line drugs before satisfactory results are obtained on DOTS implementation until results from pilot DOTS plus programs are available.

For the Bank and Other Stakeholders

1) **Regional Workshops.** The HIV/AIDS and TB Country Profiles, and the Central Asia AIDS and TB studies should be presented and discussed in regional workshops with stakeholders, including regional Governments and partner organizations.

2) **Advocacy, Communication, and Stakeholder Participation.** There is a need to improve coordination among all stakeholders involved in control of HIV/AIDS, STIs, and TB in Central Asia. In addition to the proposed regional workshops, the Bank and other stakeholders should assist regional Governments carrying out other advocacy and communication activities that will involve all stakeholders, and that will contribute to political and social consensus that ensures early adoption of effective strategies to prevent and control HIV/AIDS, STIs, and TB in Central Asia. Clearly, a multi-sectoral approach will be needed to address the dual epidemics of HIV/AIDS and TB. To reach stakeholders across sectors, an extensive communication strategy is needed. Barriers to multi-sectoral cooperation include stigma, which is notably evident in the sub region. Key sectors include health, education, military, prisons and labor. All of these have been addressed effectively in other HIV/AIDS and TB prevention efforts in other regions, and there is sufficient evidence to consider similar approaches in Central Asia.

3) **Capacity building.** In particular, training in technical areas is needed in the sub region. For example, training of laboratory technicians to be better able to identify MDRTB; training of primary care physicians to recognize, treat, and appropriately refer TB patients; training of health care providers to treat People Living with HIV/AIDS (PLWHA) with dignity in accord with human rights; training of educators to explain appropriate risks for HIV; and training of public health nurses to conduct VCT among highly vulnerable groups. Training on new screening methods for HIV will need to be done in the future as these technologies are developed and disseminated.

4) **Technical Assistance and Lending.** In the context of sector work and Bank-financed operations in the health sector and other sectors, the Bank will continue to assist regional Governments in adopting and satisfactorily implementing HIV/AIDS, STIs, and TB Strategies. In Kazakhstan, the proposed reviews of the HIV/AIDS and TB programs should be concluded.[6] In Kyrgyz Republic, the Bank should continue carrying out sector work and assisting the implementation of the Health II Project, and explore the possibility of preparing an HIV/AIDS project funded by an IDA grant. In Tajikistan, initial work to prepare an HIV/AIDS project or component, also funded by an IDA grant, has already started and should be continued in cooperation with the implementation of the GFATM grant. In Turkmenistan, the Bank should continue to track trends in drug use, HIV/AIDS, STIs, and TB, and follow up on the work carried out by the Government, UNAIDS-TG, and partner organizations to prevent and control these diseases. In Uzbekistan, the Bank

---

6. The World Bank (draft under review). ESW Concept Note on Insurance, HIV/AIDS and TB Sector Work. Washington DC: The World Bank. ECSHD.

should continue to assist the Government in preparing and implementing an HIV/AIDS operation funded by an IDA grant, and continue supporting TB activities in the country.[7]

Recommendations for Additional Studies

1) **HIV/AIDS.** The Bank is preparing for publication the Central Asia HIV/AIDS study, which aims to identify strategies to ensure early and effective interventions to control the epidemic at national and regional levels. These efforts are based on global evidence and include local partners. The study also aims to inform the Bank's policy dialogue and operational research on HIV/AIDS in Central Asia, while supporting the regional partnerships between Governments, civil society, UN agencies, and multilateral and bilateral agencies to prevent HIV/AIDS, STIs, and TB. The following specific studies were carried out as part of this activity:

   (i) **Estimate the potential impact of the HIV/AIDS epidemic in Central Asia.** This study estimates the potential epidemiological and economic impact of the HIV/AIDS epidemic in Central Asia. Most stakeholders agreed that the Bank would add value to the knowledge base by modeling the epidemic in this way. The model explores several possible scenarios that would inform discussions with stakeholders about the potential impact of the epidemic. This will serve to achieve political and social consensus to take early and effective action on the nascent epidemic in the sub region.

   (ii) **Identify gaps in strategies, policies, and legislation aimed at controlling the epidemic.** This study further the analyses in the Country Profiles and, as much as possible, estimates funding needs for implementation. It will generate recommendations for further policy development, and particular attention is paid to prison populations.

   (iii) **Identify key stakeholders.** This study identifies key stakeholders and their roles in controlling the epidemic; it describes how to increase partnership and ownership of HIV/AIDS Strategies.

   (iv) **Assess institutional capacity.** This study assesses the institutional capacity of public health services and relevant NGOs to tackle the epidemic. It is complemented by an in-depth review of the HIV/AIDS and TB Programs in Kazakhstan.

   (v) **Develop a communication and participation plan on HIV/AIDS in Central Asia.** This plan defines a communication strategy for the Bank and other interested stakeholders regarding HIV/AIDS in the sub region. The communication strategy would help create a political and social consensus that ensures early adoption of effective HIV/AIDS prevention and control strategies by Governments and other key stakeholders.

2) **TB Study.** The Bank has decided to carry out a TB Study, due to the importance of this epidemic in itself and the links between the TB and HIV/AIDS epidemics. Again, particular attention will be paid to prison populations.

3) **Drug Abuse.** The drug abuse epidemic is well established in Central Asia. In 2002, the Soros Foundation/OSI published a comprehensive study about counter-narcotics efforts in Afghanistan and Central Asia (Lubin etal. 2002). This effort should be pursued in the future to track trends in trafficking and consumption of drugs in the region, which fuels epidemics of drug use and HIV/AIDS, and contributes to the global TB epidemic. In particular, evaluation studies of harm reduction approaches are needed.

4) **Public Health System Needs.** The Bank or other stakeholders should carry out a complete assessment of HIV/AIDS, STI, and TB surveillance in Central Asia. Although

---

7. The World Bank (draft under preparation). Project Concept Document. Washington DC : The World Bank. ECSHD.

USAID/CAR, through CDC and Project HOPE, is providing significant financial and technical support to upgrading epidemiological surveillance, no comprehensive review of the existing systems is yet available. In particular, attention should be paid to behavioral surveillance, which is lacking in most of the Central Asian countries. The Bank and its clients should address the integration of public health approaches to HIV/AIDS through health systems projects, either as stand alone activities or as part of specific outcome measures for health systems development.

5) **Funding of HIV/AIDS, STI, and TB Programs in Central Asia**. The Country Profiles offer limited information regarding funding of the HIV/AIDS, STI, and TB Programs in Central Asia. However, it is expected that the proposed in-depth review of the Kazakh HIV/AIDS and TB programs, which are being carried out in the context of additional sector work co-financed by the Government of Kazakhstan and the Bank, will provide a case study of financing of HIV/AIDS and TB in the sub region.

CHAPTER I

HIV/AIDS AND TUBERCULOSIS GLOBALLY

The HIV/AIDS epidemic is spreading throughout the world with ferocious speed. HIV has infected more than 60 million people worldwide. More than 20 million have died from AIDS, with 3 million dying in 2000 alone (Table 7). There were around 40 million people living with HIV/AIDS at the end of 2002. Approximately 14,000 new infections occur each day, more than half are among those below age 25. Over 95 percent of PLWHA are in low and middle-income countries. In Sub-Saharan Africa, HIV/AIDS is now the leading cause of death, and it is the fourth biggest killer globally. In several nations, life expectancy has been cut by more than 10 years.

In addition, two billion people worldwide are infected with *Mycobactrium Tuberculosis,* an infectious agent that can lead to active TB. There are an estimated 17 million cases of active TB globally. Every year, about 9 million people develop active TB and 2 million die of the disease; 84 percent of all TB sufferers live in developing countries. Most are poor people aged between 15 to 54 years of age. Between 2000 and 2020, nearly 1 billion additional people will be infected with TB, 200 million will become sick, and 35 million will die of the disease, unless current efforts to control TB are greatly strengthened and expanded. Drug resistant TB is on the rise, greatly increasing the cost of treatment. MDRTB has already been identified in over 100 countries and more than 400,000 estimated new cases of MDRTB will develop each year. These MDRTB cases are hundred times more expensive to treat than non-resistant TB.

The countries of Central Asia are still at the earliest stages of an HIV/AIDS epidemic. Kazakhstan, the worst affected country in Central Asia, has less than 4,000 estimated HIV cases.

TABLE 7. HIV/AIDS AND TB WORLDWIDE IN 2000			
	Deaths per year	**New cases per year**	**Developing countries**
HIV/AIDS	3.0 million	5.3 million	92%
Tuberculosis	1.9 million	8.8 million	84%

Until recently, the Kyrgyz Republic, Tajikistan, Turkmenistan, and Uzbekistan were scarcely affected by HIV. However, by the end of 2002, almost 6,000 HIV-infected persons had been reported in the five republics. The main cause for serious concern is the drug trafficking routes that pass through Central Asia. These have facilitated the growth of IV drug use in the sub region; expert estimates indicate that the region may have more than 0.5 million drug users, and outbreaks of HIV-related injecting drug use have been reported in Kazakhstan, Kyrgyz Republic, Uzbekistan, and Tajikistan. Clearly, the risk of a shift in the HIV/AIDS epidemic exists in this sub region because of the risky behavior reported by IDUs and because of the increases in STIs, CSWs, migration, and other risk factors. The epidemic is currently concentrated among IDUs and CSWs, but it can and likely will spread to vulnerable groups such as young people, mobile populations, and sex partners of high-risk group members.

CHAPTER 2

HIV/AIDS AND TUBERCULOSIS IN EASTERN EUROPE AND CENTRAL ASIA

In Eastern Europe and Central Asia, HIV incidence is rising faster than in any other region of the world. The world's steepest HIV curve in 1999 was recorded in the Russian Federation, where the proportion of the population living with HIV doubled between end-1997 and end-1999. In seven years, the number of cases increased over 30 times. In 1994, there were approximately 30,000 people living with HIV/AIDS in Eastern Europe and Central Asia out of a total population of 450 million. By the end of 1999, there were an estimated 420,000 adults and children living with HIV/AIDS in Eastern Europe and Central Asia. In 2001, there were an estimated 250,000 new infections in the region, raising the number of people living with HIV/AIDS to 1 million. Over 13,000 people have developed AIDS, and over 5,000 have already died. While national rates of adult prevalence – less than one percent of the general population – are considered low by international standards, the particularly disturbing aspect is the high rate of increase in cases over recent years. Ukraine, the Russian Federation, Belarus, and Moldova have the highest numbers of people living with HIV/AIDS in the region. In Estonia, reported HIV infections have soared from 12 in 1999 to 1,112 in the first nine months of 2001.

Government officials recognize that the official statistics grossly underestimate the real prevalence of HIV. According to local and international experts the HIV/AIDS prevalence is at least ten times higher than official reports. Accurate estimates are problematic, however, because of the lack of proper epidemiological surveillance and the repressive practices of law enforcement bodies used against highly vulnerable groups.

In 2000, approximately 380,000 cases of tuberculosis (10 percent of the global TB burden) were reported in Europe, with large variation among three areas:

- 13 cases per 100,000 population in Western countries (the 15 countries of the European Union, Andorra, Iceland, Israel, Malta, Monaco, Norway, San Marino and Switzerland);
- 40 cases per 100,000 in Central European countries (Albania, Bosnia-Herzegovina, Bulgaria, Croatia, Czech Republic, Hungary, FYR of Macedonia, Poland, Romania, Slovakia, Slovenia, Turkey, and Yugoslavia); and
- 92 cases per 100,000 in the 15 countries of the Former Soviet Union (FSU).

In 1999, age-specific rates were highest among those over 64 years old in Western countries, among those 45–54 years old in Central Europe, and among those 25–34 years old in the FSU. Rates were highest among men, with greater sex differences in countries with higher reporting rates. Among cases never treated, the proportion of multi-drug resistant (MDR) cases was 0.5 percent in 18 countries in Western and Central Europe countries (range 0–2.1 percent), but it was much higher in Estonia (17.5 percent), Latvia (10.4), and Lithuania (7.8). Among cases previously treated, 3.9 percent were MDRTB in Western and Central European countries and 37 percent in the Baltic countries.

In most Western and Central European countries, stable or decreasing TB reporting rates and low levels of drug resistance indicate that TB control remains overall effective. In Western countries, cases of foreign origin represent a high and increasing proportion of TB cases. By contrast, in the FSU, the 61 percent increase in TB reporting rates between 1995 and 2000 suggests increasing TB incidence, but in some countries it may also indicate improved reporting. Increasing incidence and high levels of drug resistance indicate a reduced performance of TB control programs in a time of socio-economic hardship. These trends and the possible impact of the spreading HIV epidemic, call for urgent action to readapt and strengthen TB control programs in the FSU.

Overlap of HIV/AIDS and TB

Because of their suppressed immune system, people co-infected with HIV and TB are many times more likely to develop active TB. In other countries affected by both epidemics, the number of TB cases has doubled and even trebled in the past decade, mainly as a result of the HIV epidemic. The number of people co-infected with TB and HIV has already soared to over 10 million worldwide. Due to the economic downturn that followed the breakup of the Former Soviet Union, the subsequent poverty, and the overcrowding in prisons, tuberculosis is becoming a communicable disease crisis in Central Asia. With the concomitant rise in multi-drug resistance and the persistent problems with inappropriate therapy, this situation has global repercussions. When MDRTB reaches a level of more than 5 percent of reported cases, this becomes a worrisome situation; in Central Asia, there are already numerous regions where this level has been reached.

Although HIV/AIDS and TB probably do not yet overlap significantly in ECA, TB is the main opportunistic disease for HIV/AIDS. Projections in Russia have shown that in the presence of a moderate HIV/AIDS epidemic, TB may become uncontrollable even in the presence of a well-designed and implemented TB program (Vinokur etal. 2001). Therefore, significant attention must be paid to TB prevention and control in the region, using good quality control and universal application of DOTS programs and, when indicated, appropriately applying DOTS Plus for MDRTB. In addition, there is a critical need to conduct surveillance of MDRTB. All of this work is especially important in prisons, where overcrowding, poor nutrition, IV drug use, and HIV/AIDS are becoming more common.

Drug Abuse

One of the results of the civil strife in Afghanistan over the last 20 years was that it became the world's largest illicit drug producer. Illegal drug trafficking continues to escalate throughout Central Asia, endangering not only the health of the local population, but also having negative consequences on the political, economic, and social stability in the region. All five Central Asian countries serve as drug trafficking routes from Afghanistan to Russia and Central and Western Europe. During 2001 alone, 8.8 tons of drugs, including 4.2 tons of heroin, were seized in Tajikistan, a 26 percent increase over 2000.

Furthermore, high rates of extreme poverty and unemployment throughout the region foster the illegal drug trade. Initially serving only as transit countries for drug smugglers, Central Asia and its young population has become a lucrative market in itself for illegal drugs. One of the most visible results of increased drug trafficking through Central Asia is the increase in IV drug addiction in the region. Local drug consumption patterns are influenced by easy access to drugs. People are switching from alcohol to heroin, which is cheaper, and heroin users are starting to switch from smoking or snorting to injection, because it is a more efficient method of drug ingestion. The retail price of a single dose of heroin in Kyrgyz Republic is as low as $.50-$1. Drug interdiction efforts are insufficient to reduce the demand for drugs. Economic development, education, and destigmatization foster a more appropriate approach to the problem of IV drug use. Unless IDUs have options for substitution therapy (such as methadone), drug addiction treatments, and harm reduction programs, little progress against this risk factor for HIV/AIDS can be expected.

HIV, IDUs, and STIs

The outbreak of HIV among IDUs derives from the high prevalence of unsafe drug injecting practices. In Kazakhstan, for example, health officials reported that injecting drug use caused 85 percent of new HIV cases. In Uzbekistan, this mode of transmission accounts for 70 percent of new HIV cases. Needle sharing as well as other unsafe practices among drug users is the main factor that drives the epidemic. As sexual transmission of HIV spreads from IDUs to the general population, the virus may penetrate all layers of society. However, the lack of awareness of the underlying risk scenario and the relatively low prevalence rates of HIV/AIDS thus far has been the main reasons for the slow response from governments in the sub region. They have simply not taken the problem as seriously as is indicated.

Most of the new infections are occurring among young men, the majority of whom are injecting drug users. Economic disparity and disadvantage often force women to become commercial sex workers, and unprotected sex places both CSWs and their partners at risk of HIV infection. Furthermore, injection drug use and commercial sex are linked as sex is often exchanged for drugs.

The heterosexual-based component of the epidemic is increasing in size, and thus signals a threat to the larger populations of Central Asian Countries. UNAIDS experts report that the male-female ratio of newly detected HIV cases has narrowed from 4:1 to 2:1, indicating that women are increasingly at risk. A growing number of female injecting drug users engage in commercial sex work, which may also provide a bridge between the high-risk and general populations. Police continue the old Soviet practice of using medical professionals to identify drug users and commercial sex workers. Marginalization of these victims, including people living with HIV/AIDS, and the costs of treatment further isolate them from medical and preventive services. Not surprisingly, mother-to-child HIV transmission is also on the rise. CSWs, whether trafficked or not, are another critical risk group pool from which spread to the general population could be anticipated.

In addition, the epidemic of STIs in the sub region is of concern. Not only does the presence of STI epidemics indicate that unprotected and probably multiple exposure risky sexual behavior is common, but ulcerative STIs such as syphilis actually facilitate HIV transmission. Therefore, it is crucial to address underlying knowledge gaps, misconceptions, and reproductive health deficiencies to prevent STIs and thereby help prevent HIV/AIDS. Kazakhstan had more than 300 cases of syphilis per 100,000 population in 2000, which is the second highest prevalence rate in the European region and reflecting a more than 30-fold increase from the early 1990s. In one study conducted by the WHO in the south of Tajikistan, it was found that 76 percent of the surveyed women had had one or more STIs.

Preventive Issues

Despite such alarming incidence rates of sexually transmitted infections, the public perception of the HIV/AIDS threat is very low, and it is commonly viewed that HIV/AIDS is a problem of foreigners and drug users only. Even health professionals do not always feel comfortable discussing HIV/AIDS prevention with their patients who might be at increased risk. Furthermore, AIDS, STIS, and TB services are generally provided through vertical program structures with little or no coordination. The WHO recommends the integration of HIV/AIDS and STIs prevention (WHO 2001), and generally only the government leaders can play such an integrative role.

However, there is still a window of opportunity to prevent the HIV/AIDS epidemic from exploding. National Governments in the sub region must express the necessary political will and take decisive action before the epidemic of HIV expands beyond the concentrated risk groups. Young people are a priority on this front. Twenty years into the epidemic, millions of young people in the sub region know little, if anything, about HIV/AIDS risks and prevention. According to UNICEF, over 50 percent of young people (aged 15–24) in many countries including Uzbekistan, have never heard of AIDS or have serious misconceptions about how HIV is transmitted. Providing young people with candid information on HIV/AIDS and life skills to avoid infection is a high priority. Unprecedented numbers of young people are not completing their secondary schooling in these countries, adding to the knowledge gap. With jobs in short supply, many are at special risk of joining groups of highly vulnerable populations by resorting to injecting drug use and regular or occasional sex work.

Government Funding and Policies of the Region

Effective HIV/AIDS awareness and prevention programs have been further hampered by a severe lack of governmental resources. International organizations ultimately provide a large share of funding for such programs, but there is a need for coordinated donor, NGO, and Government activities in order to make the best use of scarce resources. With only the scarce resources available for health care, the sub region simply cannot afford the epidemic. For example, among the Central Asian states, only Kazakhstan has offered limited antiretroviral treatment to a few privileged patients. The treatment of opportunistic diseases associated with AIDS would be an additional burden for national health budgets, and in combination with ongoing epidemics of tuberculosis and STIs, such economic burdens may erase any modest economic gains made since the breakup of the FSU. Collective regional efforts with an emphasis on prevention and reduction of drug addiction are urgently needed.

All five countries have recognized the impending danger of an HIV epidemic, and have recently approved national programs on HIV/AIDS. Governments have taken positive steps to modify existing legislation to include HIV/AIDS detection and confidentiality provisions. Despite growing emphasis on a coordinated regional response, it is clear that any HIV/AIDS initiative in Central Asia must confront a cultural reluctance to confront HIV/AIDS, drug use, and sexuality. Historically, national HIV/AIDS Centers in the former Soviet Union focused on mandatory mass screening, based on traditional "identify and control the carrier" approaches. Those living with HIV/AIDS were afraid to seek treatment, fearing official and unofficial stigmatization; these fears and responses are unchanged today.

In June 2001, the Central Asian Conference on the Prevention of HIV/AIDS held in Almaty, Kazakhstan, brought together government officials, UN specialized agencies, and NGOs to discuss the explosive growth of HIV/AIDS prevalence in the region. It was the first time that Central Asian Governments openly acknowledged the problem and signed a declaration that calls for the establishment of a regional strategy to combat HIV/AIDS. The declaration is considered a major breakthrough in marking the end of the "denial era."

An effective response requires comprehensive and multi-sectoral approaches. Efforts must be made to address the socio-economic determinants of the epidemic, thereby reducing the vulnerability to drug abuse, HIV and other sexually transmitted infections. There is an urgent need to reduce the demand for and supply of drugs, particularly among young people, and to promote safer sexual behaviors. For the larger population that does not inject drugs, complementary strategies are required to prevent the spread of HIV from their high-risk sexual partners. Strategies include HIV education for injecting drug users and their partners, access to high-quality condoms and syringes, access to bleach for sterilization of injecting equipment (though recent evidence does not support this intervention), and drug treatment programs. Kazakhstan, Kyrgyz Republic, Tajikistan, Turkmenistan, and Uzbekistan are faced with a unique opportunity to intervene early and decisively to prevent the HIV epidemic from spreading from highly vulnerable groups to youth in general.

Issues Regarding TB and MDRTB

In contrast, TB is a well-established epidemic throughout the sub region. Because of the critical nature of the MDRTB component of this epidemic, it has global significance. With pockets of MDRTB prevalence reaching more than 30 percent, the global danger of spreading resistant TB throughout ECA and beyond is of concern to all donors. Some of the most important issues for decision makers involved in this problem are: (i) there is an unwillingness or lack of ability of Governments to allocate the necessary funding for DOTS implementation at the national level, including in prisons; (ii) there is inefficiency in utilization of available public resources and donor funding; and (iii) The treatment of MDRTB in Kazakhstan and Kyrgyz Republic before satisfactory DOTS implementation is ill-advised. This last statement reflects the fact that DOTS is not implemented sufficiently to provide adequate attention to the basic TB epidemic.

There are persistent therapeutic and diagnostic holdovers from the Soviet era, specifically, mass x-ray screening (MMR), which consume enormous resources without the benefit of evidence and divert attention from the proved approach of DOTS. In Uzbekistan, only 7 percent coverage of DOTS is reported (Cox and Hargraves 2003), and the case detection target of 70 percent in this country will not be reached for at least a decade. Deteriorating health systems contribute to the lack of DOTS coverage, as patients move into and out of care without the public health infrastructure necessary to sustain treatment throughout the initial course. What to do about those who have been in partial treatment (for example, for only one month) is controversial, especially since second line drugs are so difficult to procure and finance. Given the intermittent drug supply in many Central Asian republics and the wide-ranging and unregulated treatment regimens, MDRTB will be an increasing problem in the sub region.

The increase in notified cases and mortality throughout the subregion, as shown in the two graphs below, is sobering to TB control specialists. Investments in quality control, training of both

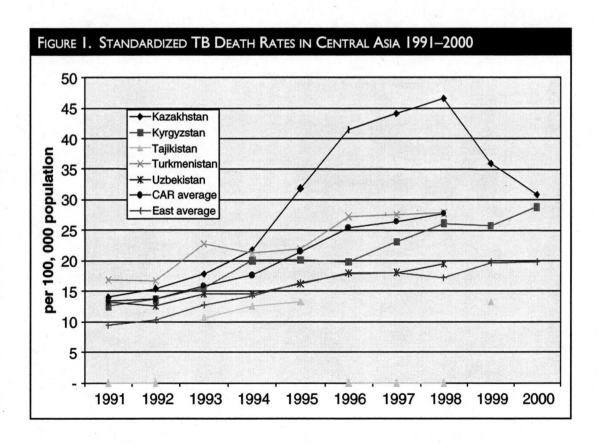

FIGURE 1. STANDARDIZED TB DEATH RATES IN CENTRAL ASIA 1991–2000

general practitioners to recognize and refer TB as well as specialists, microscopists, and clinicians to fully implement DOTS are essential and are specific needs in the sub region. These investments are very appropriate for the World Bank, but more importantly, the Bank should have a series of dialogues with country TB leaders to gain agreement on the approach to implementing DOTS and deferring second line treatments. This dialogue should involve the major bilateral donors and multilateral organizations in the sub region (especially USAID, DFID, MSF, Soros Foundation/OSI, and the WHO) to achieve consensus. Soviet-style mass screening, surgical approaches, and investments in tomography or other non-essential technology should be discouraged in the face of this dialogue on DOTS. Investments in laboratories, prison release systems that sustain DOTS, and nutritional programs will be more appropriate for the Bank and its partners. Stakeholder analysis is essential to understand how to mobilize the various sectors better, and policy analysis is essential to design culturally and nationally specific policy changes to support proved prevention approaches in Central Asia. There is much to be learned from the epidemics of HIV and TB elsewhere in the world, but there is much to be learned from local counterparts on how these evidence-based approaches can be applied in this sub region.

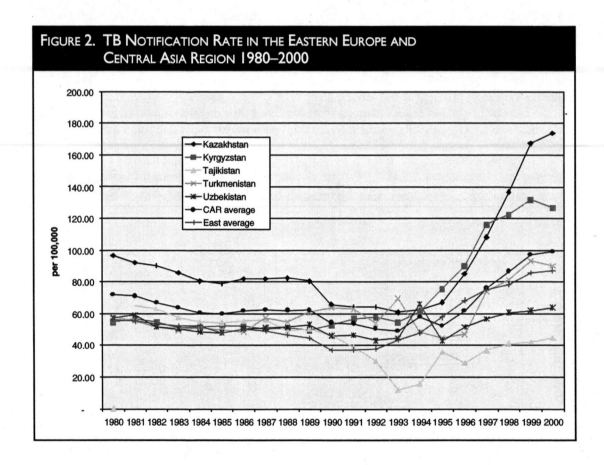

FIGURE 2. TB NOTIFICATION RATE IN THE EASTERN EUROPE AND CENTRAL ASIA REGION 1980–2000

CHAPTER 3

THE BANK'S ROLE ON HIV/AIDS AND TUBERCULOSIS IN CENTRAL ASIA

There is strong indication that the HIV epidemic is increasing in the Central Asian Republics, and it may eventually overlap with the existing TB epidemic. The HIV/AIDS and STIs epidemics mainly affect young people, while the TB epidemic affects people in their more economically productive years. This epidemiological situation may have a catastrophic impact at the household level, a significant impact on health care expenditures, and even an impact at the macroeconomic level. Therefore, the Bank decided to carry out a study of the situation in Central Asia that would review available data and evidence, gather some original data and make projections, discuss the issues with the different stakeholders, and make proposals for action. Last year, the Bank prepared a Note on HIV/AIDS in Central Asia, which was updated and posted on the ECA website.[8] This was prepared as a briefing document for the visit of the World Bank President to Central Asia, during which he agreed with regional Governments that HIV/AIDS would be one of the three priority areas for the Bank's work in the region, along with water and energy. Following this initial work, the Country and Sector Units agreed to carry out the Central Asia HIV/AIDS and TB Country Profiles and additional studies on AIDS.

The Central Asia HIV/AIDS and TB Country Profiles were developed to inform Bank management and other stakeholders about the main characteristics of the epidemics in Central Asia; differences among the countries; and main efforts to prevent HIV/AIDS and control TB. The Country Profiles summarize the information available from regional Governments and partner organizations such as UN agencies, USAID, and the Soros Foundation/OSI regarding the following aspects: epidemiology; strategic and regulatory framework; surveillance; vulnerable groups; preventive, diagnostic and treatment activities; NGO and partner activities; and funding available . The Country Profiles are based on review of existing statistics and reports and on discussions with key stakeholders, including Governments, donors, and NGOS, during missions to Central Asia.

Additional studies focusing on HIV/AIDS aim at identifying strategies for ensuring early and effective intervention to control the epidemic at national and regional levels, considering priorities

---

8. www.worldbank.org/eca/ecshd or www.worldbank.org/eca/aids.

based on global evidence. The studies also aim at informing the Bank's policy dialogue and the operational work to control HIV/AIDS in Central Asia; and contributing to building up the regional partnership between Governments, civil society, UN agencies, and multilateral and bilateral agencies to prevent HIV/AIDS and STIs. Specifically, the additional studies aim to:

   (vi) Estimate the potential epidemiological and economic impact of the HIV/AIDS epidemic in Central Asia;

  (vii) Identify key stakeholders and their roles in controlling the epidemic;

 (viii) Identify gaps in strategies, policies, and legislation aimed at controlling the epidemic;

  (ix) Assess the institutional capacity, including of public health services and NGOs, to control the epidemic; and

   (x) Prepare the Bank's communication strategy on HIV/AIDS in Central Asia.

In addition to these regional studies, the Bank has been providing technical and financial assistance to Central Asian Governments to carry out sector work and operations that tackle HIV/AIDS, STIs, and TB. The Bank has been participating in the regional HIV/AIDS work as a member of the UNAIDS-TGs, and it chairs the TG in Uzbekistan. The Bank has also been assisting some of the countries in obtaining funding to tackle the epidemic, having reviewed the GFATM grant proposals prepared by Kazakhstan and the Kyrgyz Republic (TB proposal). In Kazakhstan, in-depth reviews of the HIV/AIDS and TB programs, including expenditures reviews, are being carried out in the context of sector work co-financed by the Government and the Bank.

On the operational front, several options have been under initial consideration, including the development of a Multi-Country HIV/AIDS Program (MAP), which was suggested by UNAIDS, and investment operations and/or components in some countries financed by IDA grants. The Bank has been assisting the Government of Uzbekistan in preparing the Health II project, which is expected to have an HIV/AIDS Component, and continued supporting for TB activities. In Tajikistan, initial work to prepare an HIV/AIDS project or component also to be funded by an IDA grant, has started, and this will continue in coordination with implementation of the GFATM grant. In the Kyrgyz Republic, the Bank will continue sector work and assist implementation of the Health II Project. It may also explore the possibility of preparing an HIV/AIDS project funded by an IDA grant. In Turkmenistan, the Bank will continue to track trends in drug use, HIV/AIDS, STIs and TB, and follow up the work carried out by the Government, UNAIDS-TG and partner organizations to prevent and control these diseases.

CHAPTER 4

COUNTRY PROFILE: KAZAKHSTAN

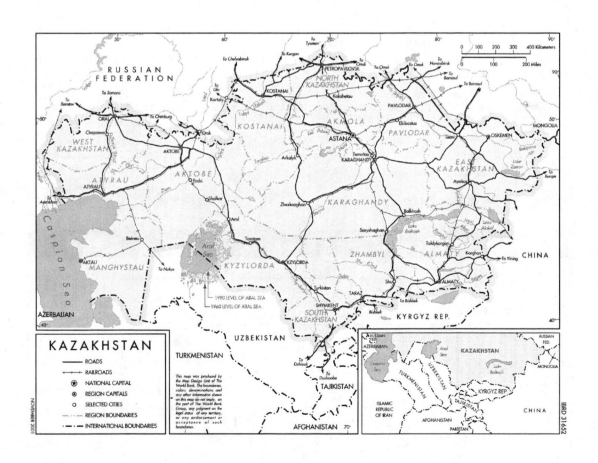

D istinguished by its large territory and relatively high annual per capita (US$1,250), Kazakhstan has a population of 15 million, of which more than 50 percent are aged 15–49 years. Approximately one-third of the population now lives below the poverty line, but 65 percent report a daily income of less than $4 per capita.

HIV/AIDS Epidemiological Profile

Kazakhstan has a reported HIV/AIDS prevalence (0.14 percent) that is higher than its four neighboring countries combined. Since the first case was reported in 1987, the number of officially reported HIV cases has grown to 3,448 by March 2003. UNAIDS experts estimate that the actual estimate is about 20,000 infected by HIV by the end of 2001. However, the Government also reported in 2002 that the incidence of HIV infection fell by 60 percent as compared with the previous year. The reasons for this reported decline are unclear, and the data require more specific investigation. It is unlikely that this reported decline can be attributed to the success of the national program, as the program has not been fully implemented as yet. It could, however, be related with use of pure heroin instead of mixtures stabilized with blood, due to the increased drug production and decreased prices.

As in most of ECA, the vulnerable groups are mainly IDUs, CSWs, prisoners, and youth in general. Factors such as poverty, high migration from neighboring areas of conflict and out of Kazakhstan, and involvement of the Army in regional peacekeeping missions increase the risks for HIV/AIDS spread. Approximately 70 percent of HIV-infected persons are aged 15–29 years; approximately 80 percent are males, although incidence is increasing among women. Official data report that 83 percent of HIV infection cases are due to risk behavior with drug injection, while sexual transmission accounts for 9 percent of the cases. Officially, in 2002, 85 people had AIDS, and 72 have died (however, UNAIDS estimates that 300 have died from AIDS). HIV-positive women have given birth to 44 infected children. Although all regions have HIV cases, the two main oblasts affected are Karaganda and Pavlodar, which account for about 70 percent of the cases.

Kazakhstan is at the center of intensive drug trafficking routes, and the number of drug users continues to increase annually. By 2002, the number of drug users registered in rehabilitation services numbered over 45,000. However, a rapid assessment response (RAR) carried out by UNAIDS in 1998–2002 suggested that the number of IDUs may exceed 250,000. According to official esti-

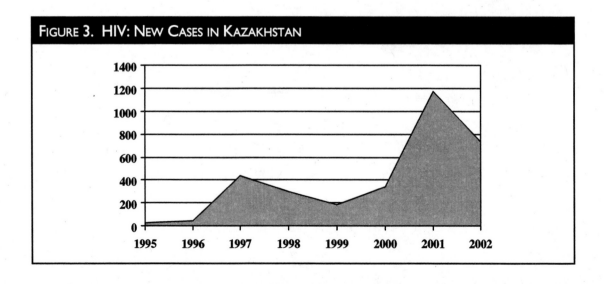

FIGURE 3.   HIV: NEW CASES IN KAZAKHSTAN

mates, 3 percent of the Kazakh population injects drugs, which would bring the number of IDUs to about 450,000. About 3–4 percent of IDUs would be infected with HIV.

The age of drug users is decreasing, and women and children are becoming active in trafficking and consumption of drugs. Now, the majority of drug users are aged 20–25 years, and 85 percent are male. Almost all drug users do not use sterilized syringes, despite considerable knowledge about risks for HIV infection. Hazardous practices such as the use of common syringes, including injecting in turns when in the company of many people, are quite common. In addition, human blood is used in the preparation of narcotics for IDU, but this practice may be decreasing, which would explain the decrease in new infections. The main drug used by IDUs is heroin, but opium is also injected. Furthermore, the majority of IDUs belong to the poorest groups, which limits their access to services including information, medical services, and clean needles.

TABLE 8. HIV/AIDS IN KAZAKHSTAN

	1990	1995	2000	2001	2002
AIDS deaths	–	3	29	57	74
AIDS cases	–	2	8	20	85
HIV cases	4	5	347	1,175	735
HIV cases among IDUs	–	3	302	1,050	
Syphilis cases	242	20,235	23,996	20,577	
Registered drug users	10,300	10,900	37,812	42,680	45,000
Registered IDUS	3,000	4,583	26,087	31,390	
Estimated # drug users	–	–	183,125	180,410	
Estimated # IDUS	–	–	130,800	128,900	250,000*
Estimated # CSW	–	–	–	13,000	50,000*
Estimated # MSM					20,000*
Trust Points (VCT)	–	–	30	96	
Harm Reduction programs	–	–	3	3	
CSW/MSM Programs	–	–	–	2	
AIDS Centers	19	19	21	21	
AIDS Centers staff	213	407	458	485	

Sources of information: Republican Center for the Prevention and Struggle Against AIDS; *UNAIDS RAR 2002

In 2002, the AIDS Center estimated there were about 20,000 MSM. In addition, approximately 20,000 to 50,000 women engaged as CSW. About 30 percent of these also use IV drugs, which they exchange for sex, and about 1 percent would be infected with HIV. The epidemic of HIV/AIDS is compounded by the spread and poor treatment of sexually transmitted infections (STIs) among these populations and subsequently in the general population. Syphilis incidence increased from less than 10/100,000 in 1986–93 to 270/100,000 in 1997; incidence gradually decreased to 160/100,000 in 2000 (UNAIDS 2002a). However, UNICEF reported STI incidence (syphilis and gonorrhea) of 320/100,000 in 2000 (UNICEF 2002), which is the highest rate among all ECA countries; this represents an increase of over 200 percent in syphilis rates since 1990 (Carinfonet 2000). According to official data of 2000, syphilis was diagnosed in 1 percent of blood donors, 1 percent of pregnant women, and 2 percent of hospital patients; in 2001, 5 percent of prisoners in temporary detention had syphilis. Data from the STI dispensaries show that 75 percent of CSW have at least one sexually transmitted disease. In 1999, more than 19,000 patients with early syphilis were placed in hospitals, accounting for over 400,000 inpatient days. The proportion of people who visited these medical providers because of syphilis was less than 30 percent, as most people can get care without being hospitalized, albeit at a great cost. Nevertheless, hospitalization for syphilis is inefficient and unnecessary with more modern practices.

Preliminary results of sentinel surveillance in selected populations show that prevalence of HIV (collected through VCT) in Karaganda is about 5 percent, in Uralsk City 2 percent and in Almaty City 0.3 percent. One study has shown that 0.5 percent of CSW were HIV positive at the end of 2001 (of 4,000 CSW screened), but the Republican AIDS Center reports that at least 1 percent of CSWs are infected. However, these data reflect high-risk group prevalence rates and not population prevalence rates.

Behavioral surveillance is important in monitoring the spread of the HIV risk factors. Surveys performed by UNAIDS show that IDUs are actually aware of HIV prevention measures: 88 percent know that single-use syringes are protective against HIV transmission, and 95 percent know that condoms can be protective. Nevertheless, many still practice unsafe IDU and have multiple casual sexual contacts without condoms; regular reported condom use does not exceed 20 percent. This is consistent with self-reported data on a history of ever having an STI (20 percent). Over half of the CSW reportedly do not use condoms, and they are not aware of other methods to prevent HIV. A survey in Almaty City has also shown that 80 percent of MSM do not use condoms, that 25 percent have had STIs, that 10 percent inject drugs, and that only 30 percent have adequate knowledge about HIV transmission These behavioral risks assure the spread of HIV from the IDU/CSW population to the general population unless effective measures are taken to reduce such risks.

It is important to understand the knowledge, attitudes, practices, and beliefs of young people in order to understand the vulnerability of this population. Interviews of school students in Almaty have shown that 13 percent of 15-year-olds have had sexual relations, 4 percent have tried drugs, 23 percent consume alcohol, and 9 percent of the sexually active have had an STI. According to the Demographic and Health Report of Kazakhstan, 17 percent of young men and 33 percent of young women aged 15–19 years do not know how to prevent HIV transmission and 27 percent of men and 65 percent of women do not use condoms during sexual intercourse with non-regular partners. UNICEF confirms that 74 percent of young men aged 15–29 and 46 percent of young women of the same age group are aware of use of condoms as a means of HIV prevention, and 54 percent of the poorest Kazakhs aged 15–49 are aware of the need to use condoms to prevent HIV transmission. In 1999, 17.5 percent of young males aged 15–24 years reported having multiple partners, while 30 percent of males and 16 percent of women aged 15–59 years reported having sex with non-regular partners; 58 percent of males and 19 percent of females aged 15–59 years reported that they used condoms (UNICEF 2002).

The prison population is of particular concern as a vulnerable population in which there are numerous risk factors for HIV and from which infected persons enter the general population (Table 9). In 2001, prisoners accounted for 25 percent of the registered HIV/AIDS cases, which

TABLE 9. PRISON POPULATIONS, FACILITIES, AND HIV PREVALENCE IN KAZAKHSTAN

	1990	1995	2000	2001
Prisoners	64,490	65,359	58,424	67,937
HIV positive	0	0	218	446
HIV prevalence (%)	0	0	0.17	0.34
People entering prisons	51,018	51,613	54,211	56,785
People released from prisons	23,895	19,354	33,222	24,544
Correctional institutions	54	60	74	75
Prisons w/ AIDS facilities				4
Prisons w/ hospitals beds				1

Sources of information: Ministry of Justice

suggests a prevalence of HIV/AIDS among prisoners of 0.5 percent, somewhat higher than officially reported. The Ministry of Justice estimates the prevalence of HIV among IDUs in prisons to be 3 percent (of 11,117 people screened). Approximately 30 percent of prisoners are IDUs, and drugs remain quite available in prisons. Injection tools are not sterilized and are used until they are completely worthless. In a study carried out in prisons, only 4 percent of the prisoners gave correct answers to questions on risks for HIV transmission and sterilization of needles. In addition, the study suggested that more than half of all prisoners have homosexual relations without condoms. There is thus a significant incidence of STIs among prisoners. Previously, prisoners were subject to obligatory tests for HIV, but this practice has been abandoned.

In summary, the HIV/AIDS epidemic in Kazakhstan is now characterized by:

- Concentration among highly vulnerable populations (IDUs, CSWs), but also spreading to other vulnerable groups (prisoners, youth, migrants, truck drivers).
- The most common mode of transmission is through the use of infected syringes and needles when injecting drugs. The potential for continued rapid spread among IDUs is enormous, as the country may have as many as 450,000 injecting drug users; their sex partners are at particular risk as well.
- Geographic concentration. The worst affected are the regions of Karaganda, Pavlodar, Kostanay, Almaty City and Uralsk City. However, all oblasts now have reported HIV cases.
- Disproportionate impact on youth, and especially young men. Over half of HIV-infected persons are aged 20–29 years. Almost 90 percent are aged 15–39 years, and about 80 percent are men.

Strategies, Policies and Legal Framework

The Government of Kazakhstan is committed to the fight against HIV/AIDS, and has recently accelerated its actions against HIV. The National HIV/AIDS Strategy, which was developed with assistance from UNAIDS, and a five-year Program were approved. The Government's National Strategy is a very thorough document, and identifies the need to raise public awareness and involve the general population, since many people including local government officials do not realize the extent of the problem. An Inter-ministerial Coordination Committee on AIDS has been established under the chairmanship of the Deputy Prime-Minister since 1995. After reconstitution, it met officially on June 11, 2002 to launch the national strategy. In addition, the Ministries of Justice and Interior have been developing their own sectoral programs.

Recently, the Government convened a Country Coordination Committee, which includes several ministries and governmental organizations, NGOs, and UN agencies, to submit a funding proposal to the GFATM. Obstacles identified by the Government include the concurrent epidemics of both injecting drug use and sexually transmitted infections; lack of social and legal tolerance for activities directed towards vulnerable populations; slow progress in changing the foci from clinical treatment methods towards promotion of healthy lifestyles and prevention activities; and insufficient resources.

The National Program has three primary objectives: to stabilize HIV prevalence by preventing the virus from spreading from highly vulnerable populations to the general population; to reduce the growth of the HIV-vulnerable sub-populations (especially youth); and to ensure that at least 80 percent of HIV-infected persons are covered with medical and social programs. To meet these objectives, the following main strategies of response against HIV were developed:

- Improving the legal basis related to HIV/AIDS. This includes strengthening measures to ensure the constitutionally guaranteed rights and freedoms of citizens, including those who engage in risky behaviors and HIV-infected persons;
- Improving national policy and practices to support relations between the Government, civil society, and groups which engage in risky behavior;

■ Developing and implementing educational programs and establishing an information environment that promotes an understanding of the HIV/AIDS issue and the hazards of risky behavior;

■ Improving the performance of health services, quality control of medical and hygienic goods, and monitoring and evaluation of the situation with respect to the HIV/AIDS epidemic;

■ Strengthening the organization of management, coordination, and performance of preventive programs on HIV/AIDS.

The Law on HIV/AIDS prevention covers the following mandates: 1) It makes the Government responsible for provision of treatment free of charge to HIV/AIDS patients and for the social protection of HIV-infected people; 2) It calls on the Government to provide information on HIV/AIDS, to carry out prevention activities, and to guarantee the human rights of people with HIV/AIDS and of risk-group members.

The National Program also addresses legal and social issues, liberalization of law enforcement practices, and mobilization of funds for the implementation of the program. For example, there is criminal punishment for the illegal purchase and storage of narcotics in large quantities. However, the President has recently commissioned a study on the experience of countries that have decriminalized 'softer drugs' and the potential ramifications of legalizing drugs such as marijuana. The grant proposal submitted to the GFATM envisages softening of the hard line approach to criminal prosecution for any procurement and storage of drugs, and allowing substitution therapy for the management of opium/heroin addiction, which is presently prohibited. Criminal and administrative prosecution for people engaging in voluntary sexual relations was recently lifted, but CSW, MSM, and people with HIV/AIDS are still highly stigmatized. Additional research, training, and public information on destigmatization are needed.

Surveillance Needs and Additional Studies

Mandatory HIV testing only applies to blood donation, organ donations, and other biological fluid transfers, but it is available on a voluntary basis for the rest of the population. Diagnosed, confirmed HIV infections are centralized into one national HIV case reporting data file, but this at present relies on passive reporting by clinical facilities; anonymous, unlinked VCT is not yet widely implemented in Kazakhstan. In the context of the USAID/ CAR HIV/AIDS Prevention Strategy, the US CDC has been assisting the Republican Center for Prevention and the Struggle Against AIDS to establish sentinel surveillance systems throughout the country in order to obtain more specific information on high-risk populations. In addition, operational research is needed to determine the efficacy of HR and outreach programs among these groups.

Vulnerable and Highly Vulnerable Groups

General knowledge on reproductive health issues in general, HIV/AIDS, and STIs is very low, as shown by behavioral surveys in both the general public and youth. According to national surveys, only 15 percent of young people have an adequate knowledge of HIV prevention, and only 10 percent of schools have integrated programs on HIV/AIDS, STIs, and drug use into their curricula. The population has a very low perceived risk of HIV infection because people do not believe that the disease will affect them personally. Currently, there are no programs on mass media regarding HIV/AIDS, but the HIV/AIDS Coordination Committee is planning to launch an information, education and communication (IEC) campaign to raise public awareness. The Ministry of Information has been given the task of developing a program and is expected to start an HIV/AIDS campaign soon. The Astana and Almaty City Healthy Lifestyle Centers are responsible for HIV/AIDS education, for example, coordinating health education activities in mass media and the education sector.

The establishment of Trust Points for IDUs and other marginalized groups may help raise the level of awareness among these highly vulnerable groups. The Trust Points are associated with harm reduction (HR) programs (education, testing, counseling, needle exchange and condom social marketing). The country has 21 AIDS centers operating in all regions and major cities. The AIDS Centers and NGOs have established 98 Trust Points, which provide highly vulnerable groups with syringes, condoms, brochures, and pre- and post-testing counseling. Trust Points use volunteers who are former drug users to provide appropriate education and information.

However, many people who are HIV-positive IDUs do not use them for fear of being harassed, and the performance of these points varies throughout the regions. For example, health professionals consider that Trust Points work well in Pavlodar, but are not very efficient in Almaty. When the centers first opened it was very difficult to establish trust in these resources among IDUs and other marginalized populations. HIV positive people were considered criminals, and in general they do not contact the AIDS Centers or NGOs for assistance. The Trust Points publicize that syringes can be exchanged anonymously, but IDUs may not yet believe this information.

Trust Points are usually located in out-patient clinics, but the AIDS Centers are planning to use other venues, such as pharmacies, to establish needle exchange programs. Furthermore, Trust Points need to be evaluated and scaled up to cover more clients. The Soros Foundation/OSI has undertaken a study to determine coverage and effectiveness of these programs for the highly vulnerable populations in Kazakhstan. In 2001, around 1 million syringes and condoms were distributed, but overall, only about 10 percent of the estimated 250,000 IDUs and 50,000 CSWs have had access to programs. A network of Narcology Dispensaries deals with treatment and rehabilitation of drug users, but these programs are not able to provide sufficient services to the growing number of IDUs, nor are they sufficiently integrated into surveillance systems or VCT programs.

Preventive, Diagnostic, and Treatment Issues
The National AIDS Center only recently established contact with Dermatology and Venereal Disease Dispensaries that provide diagnosis and treatment of STIs. However, there are numerous problems in providing services to highly vulnerable populations such as CSWs and to vulnerable populations such as youth through such institutions. In addition, they do not yet coordinate activities with the AIDS centers and other organizations working on HIV/AIDS prevention. In 1999, more than 19,000 patients with early syphilis were placed in hospitals, accounting for over 400,000 inpatient days, leading to millions of dollars of unnecessary health care costs. According to international protocols, patients only need outpatient treatment for primary and secondary syphilis. In 1999, the proportion of syphilis patients who visited these dispensaries was estimated to be less than 30 percent; many patients obtain anonymous care without hospitalization, albeit at a great cost to themselves individually. When this care is provided outside of the public health system, it represents a major deficiency in the approach to coordinated treatment of STIs. The public health approach requires contact tracing and treatment, and it also can provide a linked approach to voluntary HIV testing for STI patients. In particular, syphilis patients are at very high risk for HIV transmission, given the lack of safe sex practices as well as the biological vulnerability created by ulcerative lesions found in syphilis.

Reproductive health services and family practice centers are also expected to have a role on HIV/AIDS prevention, but again, integration and coordination with the national program are lacking. With USAID support, PSI has launched a program, "Social marketing for preventive maintenance of HIV infection and venereal diseases." Under this program, about five million condoms are being delivered to Kazakhstan. A portion of these will be distributed free of charge among groups of risk, and others will be distributed through drugstores. The project is estimated to cost US$1.5 million over two years.

In terms of treatment, hospitals, TB centers, and oncological dispensaries are expected to provide treatment for AIDS opportunistic diseases and palliative care for terminal cases. Anti-retroviral drugs are very expensive and treatment is not free. Only children under 15 years of age and infected pregnant women have access to anti-retroviral treatment under the public-financed health system.

NGO and Partner Activities

The Government intends to increase the participation of civil society, including NGOs and the private sector, in the implementation of the HIV/AIDS Program. However, the Government is not yet allowed to contract NGOs to carry out work with vulnerable and highly vulnerable groups, which has been undertaken by the AIDS Center with support from UN agencies and international NGOs such as Soros Foundation/OSI. However, the MoH recently contacted two local NGOs (Equal to Equal and East to West) to discuss cooperation between AIDS Centers and NGOs. The local NGOs would like to have a forum to improve communication and cooperation among these organizations, but funding for such coordination is lacking. All UN agencies have assisted the Government of Kazakhstan, technically and financially, in implementing HIV/AIDS prevention activities. In particular, UNAIDS has been assisting the Government of Kazakhstan on policy issues. The Bank and the Government are carrying out a review of the HIV/AIDS and STIs services under a sector study jointly financed by the Government and the Bank. According to other partners and NGOs, the Bank could have a potential role in carrying out epidemiological and economic projections of the epidemic, and assisting the development of STI case management and clinical protocols for prevention and treatment of HIV/AIDS. The procurement of pharmaceuticals was also mentioned as an area that needs further financial support.

Funding

In 2001, the Government allocated about $370 million to the health sector (about $25 per capita per year), and out-of-pocket expenses for the population were $28 million (about $2 per capita per year). The Government estimates the costs of the HIV/AIDS Program at about $150 million for the period 2001–2005. In 2001, the Government allocated $2.5 million to the implementation of the HIV/AIDS Program, and in 2002 $2.7 million. However, funding is not actually disbursed, and most of the AIDS regional centers carry out their prevention programs through grants from NGOs and bilateral organizations. The Government estimates that about $11 million will be available from different sources for HIV/AIDS control in the next three years, but additional funding is necessary in 2002–2007. Therefore, the Government, through the Coordinating Committee, has submitted a grant proposal to the GFATM in the amount of $23 million for HIV/AIDS and an additional $4.5 million for HIV/TB for the coming five years. The Global Fund has approved $6.5 million for the initial two years.

NGOs and other multi-national organizations have also provided significant programmatic funding for HIV/AIDS prevention. UN agencies finance approximately $830,000 worth of HIV/AIDS prevention and healthy lifestyles programs. Soros Foundation/OSI has invested $600,000 in harm reduction programs in 1998–2001, and this helps support more than 90 Trust Points in 2002. These prevention programs are expanding nationwide. USAID provides a $6.7 million prevention program in Kazakhstan, in the context of which the CDC is helping to develop sentinel surveillance activities. This includes substantial training to improve data collection, management, and behavioral surveillance. Population Services International carries out condom social marketing and IEC. UNICEF has been carrying out a $4.5 million program for 2000–2004 to support children and youth health activities, including HIV/AIDS prevention and education.

Tuberculosis Epidemiological Profile

Kazakhstan bears one of the greatest burdens of TB in the Central Asian region; at the end of 2001 there were 48,701 registered cases with active TB. Each year, 20–25,000 people get TB, and 4–6,000 die of TB. Between 1990 and 2001, reported rates of new TB cases and deaths in Kazakhstan increased 2.4 times (Table 10). Prevalence of TB varied from 121/100,000 population to 308/100,000 across Kazakh oblasts (Table 12). Following the successful implementation of a national DOTS strategy (since 1998), the treatment success rate increased to 83 percent in 1999 and 2000, and the TB death rate declined 36 percent in 2001 from its peak in 1998. The growth rate of new TB cases slowed significantly since 1998, although the rate reported in 2001 remained

TABLE 10. TUBERCULOSIS RATES, KAZAKHSTAN
(per 100,000 civilian population)

	1990	1995	1996	1997	1998	1999	2000	2001
Mortality	10.1	26.4	34.6	37.7	38.4	30.7	26.4	24.5
Prevalence	270.4	235.9					301.2	328.4
Case notification rate	65.8	67.1	82.5	91.3	118.4	141	153.2	155.7
Among children	23.2	20					50.9	48.4
% smear (+) cases	31	31					39	39

Source: Ministry of Health

TABLE 11. TUBERCULOSIS IN PRISONS, KAZAKHSTAN
(Absolute numbers and rates per 100,000)

	1997	1998	1999	2000	2001
TB deaths	1,302	1,218	345	175	174
TB mortality rate	880	820	300	140	130
TB prevalence	11,903	12,970	13,697	10,061	8,060
New TB cases	5,555	5,061	5,591	3,434	3,038
TB notification rate	5,591	4,268	2,995	2,515	2,210

Source: CDC (2002) Central Asia Infectious Disease Network.

the highest in the sub-region. USAID/CDC estimates that the implementation of the DOTS strategy in Kazakhstan saved approximately 13,000 lives during the period 1998–2001.

Due to overcrowding and poor ventilation and nutrition in the prisons, reported TB incidence and mortality rates were significantly higher in the prison sector than in the general population (30 and 9 times, respectively) (Table 11). However these figures represent a significant improvement since 1997. Reporting and death rates in the prisons declined 61 percent and 85 percent, respectively. The Ministry of Justice, which administers the prisons, interprets such a positive change as the result of the implementation of the DOTS approach in the prison system.

While Kazakhstan has successfully introduced and is currently implementing the DOTS strategy, multi-drug resistant tuberculosis (MDRTB) remains of great public health concern. Although there have not been national data available on drug resistance, resistance is estimated to be around 10 percent of all smear positive cases. The WHO and International Union Against Tuberculosis and Lung Diseases (IUATLD) qualify countries and regions as MDRTB hot spot areas if the rate exceeds 5 percent. Data from the National Reference Laboratory for 2000 indicate that the rates of multi-drug resistance vary between 9 to 22 percent among the Regions with sufficient surveillance data (Table 13). The surveillance system will expand to improve this information on a national level.

TABLE 12. TB PREVALENCE RATES BY OBLAST
(per 100,000 population)

Oblast	2000
Almaty	121–146
Almaty City	121–146
Northern Kazak	121–146
Southern Kazak	121–146
Eastern Kazak	121–146
Karaganda	121–146
Kostanay	121–146
Astana City	147–173
Akmola	147–173
Jambyl	147–173
Atyrau	174–200
Western Kazak	174–200
Pavlodar	174–200
Aktubinsk	201–226
Mangistau	227–281
Kyzylarda	281–308

Source: CDC Central Asia Infectious disease network, 2002

Strategies, Policies, and Legal Framework

Government commitment to TB control is significant, as demonstrated by the following activities:

- Kazakhstan has a National TB control program based on the WHO recommended TB control strategy, DOTS, 'adjusted to Kazakhstan conditions,' which covers the entire population;
- Procurement of TB drugs is centralized at the national level;
- There is no shortage of first line drugs across the entire nation.

In May 1998, President Nasarbayev of Kazakhstan issued an order calling for the nationwide implementation of DOTS and allocating a state budget for procurement of TB pharmaceuticals. The needs for first line TB drugs are identified at six-month intervals by monitoring the stock of drugs in each facility through a nationwide computerized system. As decreed by the President, the Government of Kazakhstan has accepted DOTS as the country's official TB control strategy. The Ministry of Health is responsible for all tuberculosis-related activities, and the TB Scientific Research Institute implements and coordinates the DOTS strategy. All DOTS programs, including those run by NGOs, are approved by the Institute before implementation.

TABLE 13. MULTIPLE-DRUG RESISTANT TUBERCULOSIS SURVEILLANCE (%), KAZAKHSTAN

Oblast	Primary		Secondary		Total	
	I drug	MDR	I drug	MDR	I drug	MDR
Almaty	45.9	9.9	66.2	12.3	58.8	11.4
Almaty City	36.5	16.2	39.9	19.2	38.9	18.2
Northern Kazak	58.1	9.8	63.6	21.8	61.4	42.3
Southern Kazak	37.1	7.5	37.8	9.2	37.7	8.9
Eastern Kazak	44.2	6.3	90.0	27.8	71.3	19.1
Karaganda	56.9	10.1	70.8	22.3	64.5	16.8
Kostanay	21.8	5.5	63.4	13.5	50.8	11.0
Astana City	72.9	13.9	87.7	48.0	39.4	5.5
Akmola	39.2	6.7	55.8	10.5	46.7	8.4
Jambyl	12.6	–	82.6	2.0	37.0	1.0
Atyrau	26.1	–	57.4	6.4	33.9	1.9
Western Kazak	86.2	10.3	87.0	14.2	87.2	13.7
Pavlodar	78.8	12.1	93.7	34.4	91.3	30.8
Aktubinsk						
Mangistau	72.2	25.9	86.8	26.2	80.0	26.1
Kyzylarda	33.0	16.8	21.1	34.3	73.6	22.9
Kazakhstan	46.2	9.7	62.7	18.3		

Source: National TB Research Institute (2002).

Surveillance Needs and Additional Studies

TB electronic surveillance allows policy makers to have reliable data, analyze trends rapidly, and make informed decisions. The TB Electronic Surveillance Case-Based Management (ESCM) System developed with assistance from the CDC became fully operational throughout the country, with a database established in January 2000 (more than 65,000 TB cases). The system is fully compatible with both WHO and Soviet surveillance systems. However, it is unclear whether the Ministry of health maintains the system or has reverted to the previous Soviet surveillance system. This system would need to be scaled up to also include resistance testing in order to determine the applicability of DOTS-Plus approaches to drug resistant TB. Additional studies are needed to determine if high rates of MDRTB and co-existing HIV infection can explain 7 to 9 percent DOTS treatment failure and 5 percent TB mortality rates.

In the context of the policy dialogue and sector work co-financed by the Government and the Bank, an in-depth review of the National TB Program is being carried out. This review includes an analysis of epidemiological data, a facilities survey and focus groups with patients and providers.

Preventive, Diagnostic, and Treatment Issues

Following the introduction of DOTS in 1998, population coverage expanded rapidly to the entire country in 2000, which had a significant effect on the TB epidemic situation in Kazakhstan. The mortality rate decreased immediately, and the growth in incidence slowed. However, treatment success is yet to reach the WHO target of 85 percent. Significant decreases in mortality and incidence as the result of DOTS implementation and coordination with the prison system emphasize the importance of uninterrupted anti-TB drug supply and treatment of released prisoners in Kazakhstan.

An issue of concern is the efficiency of the utilization of available resources and donor funding. Although the Kazakhstan National TB Program claims adherence to the DOTS strategy, including passive case detection by sputum microscopy, X-ray mass screening is still excessively and inappropriately applied (Table 14). In 2001, approximately two-thirds of the entire adult population was screened through more than 5 million MMRs (mass screening by miniature radiography -fluorography). This amounted to 517 MMRs per TB case detected. Thirty digital fluorography machines were procured in 2001. With similar treatment success rates in Kazakhstan and Kyrgyz Republic, average length of hospital stay per patient treated is noticeably higher in Kazakhstan than in Kyrgyz Republic, 92 and 74 days respectively, suggesting significant over-utilization of hospital-based facilities in Kazakhstan.

TABLE 14. TB SERVICE PROVISION, KAZAKHSTAN

	1990	1995	2000	2001
TB facilities	350	345	341	334
Sanatoria	39	34	30	32
TB offices/ posts in general health care facilities	127	136	159	147
TB beds	19,815	15,733	13,490	13,522
Sanatoria beds	5,925	4,541	3,843	4,040
TB physicians	1,522	1,280	1,305	1,346
Inpatient days (thousands)	5,787	4,674	4,329	4,477
Average length of stay	128	120	97	92
Surgeries		199	1,255	1,565
Fluorography machines	604	659	545	601
Digital Fluorography machines				30
Screening radiography tests (MMR)	6,965	6,803	3,892	5,177
% population that underwent screening radiography tests	42	41	26	35
BCG vaccinations and revaccinations (thousands)	662.8	698.7	404.8	411.3
Sputum smears for detection of TB (thousands)			1046.6	1016.9
Sputum culture tests (thousands)			334.9	261.1
Sputum DST (drug susceptibility tests) for TB			10,001	11,107

Source: Ministry of Health

There is no nationwide program to control MDRTB in Kazakhstan as yet. There is evidence that 60 to 80 percent of MDRTB patients can be cured with appropriate management based on second- and third-line drugs (DOTS-Plus). Appropriate integration of the DOTS-Plus strategy into the National TB program in Kazakhstan appears to be justified. Concerned with the magnitude of the MDRTB problem and its outcome, the Government has taken the following actions: (i) established four pilot sites for DOTS-Plus (USAID/CAR, through Project Hope and CDC, developed two additional pilots); (ii) developed an application to the WHO Green Light Committee for procurement of second-line drugs at lower cost; and (iii) used a World Bank loan to purchase TB drugs, transportation vehicles for oblast TB dispensaries, laboratory equipment and supplies, and the national TB reference lab with full capacity for TB drug-susceptibility testing.

The four pilot sites (North Kazakhstan and South Kazakhstan Oblasts, Almaty City, and the National TB Center) now provide diagnosis and treatment of MDRTB, and they collectively followed a total of 300 patients in 2000. In 2001, two more pilots were established for MDRTB treatment (Aktubinsk and Karaganda Oblasts) with USAID assistance, increasing the number of followed patients to 400 in 2001. In 2002, the Government provided second line drugs to six more oblasts (East Kazakhstan, Zhambyl, West Kazakhstan, Kzyl-Orda, Mangistay and Pavlodar), covering 1,300 more patients for MDRTB. In 2003, the Government plans to expand MDRTB treatment to the entire country.

Since 2000, the Government has been purchasing second-line drugs for the pilot projects. However, the rapid expansion of the MDRTB treatment programs lacks appropriate clinician training, laboratory capacity for drug susceptibility testing, and proceeds good implementation of standard DOTS protocols. Therefore, the possible establishment of resistance to second-line drugs is a cause of concern. One of the most important issues is the lack of scientifically validated treatment protocols used by Kazakh physicians and the lack of local technical capacity to deal with MDRTB.

NGO and Partner Activities

The National TB Program started at the end of 1999 with World Bank support. Its aims are to improve treatment and strengthen policy reform and management of TB control throughout the Republic. The WHO provided technical assistance to this Bank-financed project. With financial and technical assistance from USAID and its implementing partners (US CDC and Project HOPE), the DOTS strategy was successfully expanded to the entire country by 2000. The Government has allocated funds for regular monitoring of DOTS implementation. Project HOPE has been providing DOTS training to both TB specialists and primary health care physicians since 1997. The CDC has been active in upgrading laboratories and improving skills of TB laboratory workers. CDC provided training on Electronic Surveillance Case-Based Management data analysis to the oblast TB dispensaries throughout the country.

Recognizing the severity of the problem in Central Asia, USAID/CAR began assisting the implementation of DOTS in four pilot sites in Kazakhstan since 1997. Following up on the Government's request in 1998, USAID expanded technical assistance to 21 pilot TB dispensaries. USAID's DOTS implementing partners are Project HOPE and CDC, which work nationwide. Project HOPE helps counterparts to develop the legal and policy framework, and helps in upgrading the skills of both TB specialists and primary health care physicians. Project HOPE is in the process of introducing standard monitoring check lists for regular DOTS implementation monitoring and evaluation in close collaboration with the Government. Recently, Project HOPE and CDC started a new TB control and prevention program in the Karaganda prison.

While continuing to consider the DOTS strategy as a top priority for action against tuberculosis in Kazakhstan, USAID/CAR recognizes that MDRTB presents a considerable threat to the effectiveness of the country's DOTS program. In order to help the Government of Kazakhstan in its MDRTB management efforts, the USAID Regional Office for Central Asia has been providing technical assistance to the establishment of a comprehensive model for management of MDRTB. This would be tested in two pilot sites based in the TB dispensaries in Almaty city and Karaganda

Oblast. The main goal of the project is to establish the most cost-effective and scientifically proven standard MDRTB treatment protocols, monitor performance at the pilot sites, provide training for the management of MDRTB, and extrapolate experience gained to the national level.

There are several NGOs involved in health care in Kazakhstan. However, there is only one national NGO involved in TB control, the Almaty Oblast Association of TB Patients (Kurmangazy, Beg-ali).

Funding

In 2001, the Government and donors allocated US$32 million to TB diagnosis and treatment, and in 2002, the Government has allocated $8 million to the procurement of first-line and second-line TB drugs. This means that Kazakhstan spends about $640 per TB patient each year, which is three times as much as that used on cost estimates of TB programs that follow the DOTS approach; and $160 per patient per year on pharmaceuticals. Of the $200 per patient per year that a DOTS program may cost, $50 would be for procurement of first-line drugs. The increasing funding that is allocated from the state budget to the TB program has become a concern to the Accounting Chamber, which was interested in having the program reviewed, including an expenditures and cost-effectiveness study.

However, more funding would be needed for expansion of DOTS in prisons and introduction of DOTS Plus in the civilian sector. Based on a TB prevalence of 153 per 100,000 population in 2000, an average national rate of MDRTB of 10 percent among smear (+) would suggest that Kazakhstan has about 2,300 MDRTB patients. MDRTB treatment costs about US$5,000 per patient in Kazakhstan, which would require about US$11.5 million annually if all MDRTB patients were treated.

In 1999, the Bank provided a loan of US$9.5 million to the Kazakh health sector. Under the project, laboratories in many parts of the country were equipped to perform TB Mycobacterium culture and reliable drug susceptibility testing. The Bank has recently agreed with the Government of Kazakhstan to co-finance health sector studies. This could include a review of the TB Program, following up on a request from the Accounting Chamber, which is concerned with the perceived high cost of the TB program and lack of significant TB control.

The Government estimates that $170 million will be available from different sources for TB control in 2003–2005. Furthermore, it has recently submitted a $31 million grant funding proposal to the Global Fund to Fight AIDS, TB and Malaria, which would allow the financing of DOTS Plus and cover all prisons with DOTS. This funding has not been granted yet.

The Government, NGOs and partner community have indicated that additional funding would be necessary for: 1) improved nutrition for TB patients; 2) raising awareness of health staff and public about TB to ensure early detection of TB cases; 3) training of general health care staff on DOTS and DOTS Plus; 4) drug resistance prevalence survey; and 5) provision of second line TB drugs and lab equipment for MDRTB diagnosis and DOTS Plus treatment monitoring (cultures and DST).

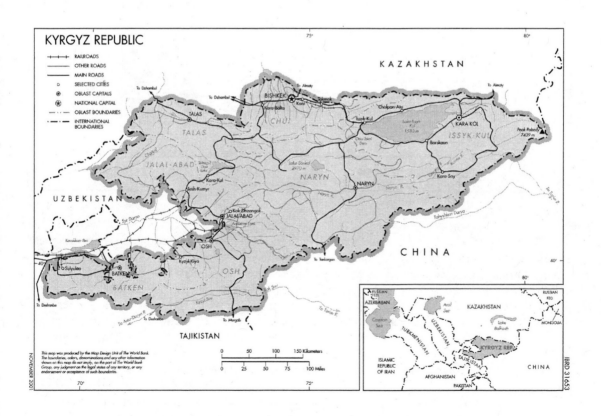

Chapter 5

Country Profile:
Kyrgyz Republic

The Kyrgyz Republic is the smallest country in Central Asia in terms of both territorial size and population (about 5 million), and one of the poorest, with US$270 per capita of annual income. More than 50 percent of the population is aged 15–49 years, and more than half live in poverty (less than US$1.00 per day).

HIV/AIDS Epidemiological Profile

The Kyrgyz Republic still has a low level of HIV prevalence. However, the country is now experiencing a rapid increase in the number of newly registered HIV-infected persons, especially over the past two years (Table 1). By May 2003, there were a total of 410 officially registered HIV cases, of which 309 were identified in 2001 and 2002. One hundred fourty nine were identified in 2001, a trebling of the total number of cases that had been identified in the period 1987–2000. However, UNAIDS estimates that the real number of HIV cases was 500 in 2001 (UNAIDS 2002b). The prevalence of HIV infection is highest among males (74 percent), especially those aged 29 years and younger (64 percent). Approximately 56 percent of cases are found among prison inmates. The worst affected region is Osh, with more than 50 percent of the cases, but Bishkek and Chui are also heavily impacted. Osh is at a crossroads of drug routes from Afghanistan to Russia. In 2001, there were four living AIDS patients with seven reported previous AIDS deaths.

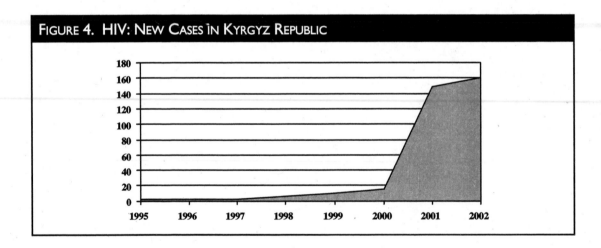

FIGURE 4. HIV: NEW CASES IN KYRGYZ REPUBLIC

The HIV/AIDS problem is closely linked with increasing drug trafficking and the consequent increase in the number of IDUs. Approximately 83 percent of cases report IDU as the main risk factor. Astonishingly, various experts estimate that about three of every four IDUs are already HIV-positive. In 2000, sentinel surveillance found an HIV prevalence of 12–19 percent among IDUs in Bishkek and 32–50 percent in Osh, which has led the MoH to estimate the number of IDUs HIV-infected in Bishkek at about 6,500, and in Osh at about 2,050. Behavioral surveys carried out in 2000 found that 96 percent of drug users share syringes, 99 percent inject drugs with a syringe from a common container, 35 percent use one syringe more than 20 times; 42 percent share syringes; 64 percent cannot afford to buy syringes; and only 14 percent use sterile syringes.

Kyrgyz has one of the largest populations of IDUs in Central Asia (an estimated 55,000, of which 65 percent are below the age of 35 years), and consequently the highest estimated population prevalence of drug users in the region (1,700–2,000/100,000).[9] The average age of drug users is

---

9. UNODCCP (UN Office for Drug Control and Crime Prevention) estimate 2001.

14 to 15 years. This situation has created a market for drug dealers, not only in the south but now in the north of the country, especially in larger cities. In 2002, only about 5,000 drug users were officially registered as patients at Narcology Centers, and almost 70 percent of these were opium users. Rates of newly registered drug users increased from over 30/100,000 in 1992 to over 100/100,000 in 1999 and from 73/100,000 in Osh to 280/100,000 in Bishkek in 1999. A dose of heroin costs 50 cents in Osh, which makes it cheaper than a bottle of vodka or even beer, and $2 in Bishkek. In a region where the average monthly salary remains below US$50, drug production and dealing are a tempting source of income in this poverty-stricken former Soviet republic. Many young Kyrgyz citizens are turning to drugs as an escape from economic hardship and lack of opportunities.

The prevalence of HIV among prisoners was 776/100,000, which is 130 times higher than among the adult population in the country. In 2001, the prevalence of syphilis among prisoners was also very high at 3,500/100,000, or 70 times higher than among the country population. About 70 percent of prisoners are drug users, and 80 percent of these are IDUs. An anonymous survey found that 40–50 percent of prisoners use injection drugs, and given the high rates of syphilis in this population, it is clear that they are also engaged in high-risk sexual behavior.

While only 4 percent of HIV cases were due to heterosexual transmission in 2001, this percentage increased to 23 percent in 2002. The HIV epidemic was preceded by a STI epidemic. In 2002, UNICEF reported that Kyrgyz Republic had one of the highest burdens of STIs in the region (almost 300/100,000 population of new cases of syphilis and gonorrhea in 2000). According to official statistics, incidence of syphilis declined from 167/100,000 population in 1997 to 73.5 in 2000, although rates still varied from 225 in Karakol City to 41 in the Djalal-Abadskaya Oblast. In addition, it is estimated that about 3,000 people are involved in sex work. Among CSWs that visited STI services in 2001, 37 percent had syphilis.

TABLE 15. HIV/AIDS, KYRGYZ REPUBLIC

	1995	2000	2001
AIDS deaths			7
AIDS cases			4
HIV estimated cases			500
HIV registered cases	17	53	149
HIV among IDUs (registered cases)		28	143
Syphilis cases		73.5	
Registered drug users	2,136	4,479	5,057
Registered IDUs	1,108	3,261	3,474
Estimated # drug users			100,000
Estimated # IDUS			55,000
Estimated # CSW			3,000
Estimated # MSM			5,000

Source: Ministry of Health

Strategies, Policies, and Legal Framework

The Kyrgyz Republic appears to be taking the threat of drugs and HIV/AIDS quite seriously, and stands out in the region as being particularly innovative in its response to the epidemics. Kyrgyz's willingness to respond to a potential HIV epidemic during the early years—when the first cases of the virus were first identified—can be considered international best practice. Although seriously under-funded, the Government has actively taken measures to address the potential epidemic with assistance from national NGOs and international partners. The HIV/AIDS Coordinating Committee is headed by the First Vice Prime Minister of Emergency Preparedness.

AIDS and prevention of STIs are both included in the Health Reform Program "Manas" and in the State Program "Healthy Nation." In 1996, when only four cases of HIV had been identified in the entire country, the Parliament adopted a Law on AIDS Prevention. The adoption of this Law undoubtedly intensified HIV prevention activities in the country, ensured the involvement of all state agencies, and facilitated securing funds for special programs. The first National Program on HIV/STIs Prevention was approved in 1997, and the "Strategic Plan of National Response to the Epidemic of HIV/AIDS in the Kyrgyz Republic" was approved in 2000. The general objective of the prevention program is to reduce the number of HIV infected people, reduce the scale of the spread of HIV, and reduce the incidence of STI incidence in the Kyrgyz Republic. Five strategies and interventions have been identified:

- Development of a national policy on HIV/AIDS and STIs;
- Ensuring the safe provision of medical procedures, including prevention of HIV and other infections through blood transmission, invasive procedures, and unsafe injection;
- Prevention of the sexual transmission of HIV and STIs, through the fostering of safe sexual behavior, the provision of condoms, and the provision of medical care for STIs;
- Prevention of the prenatal transmission of HIV by providing the population group of fertile age with information on HIV/AIDS and STIs regarding family planning, and the provision of condoms; and
- Provision of medical and social care for HIV-positive patients, AIDS patients, and their family members.

The decriminalization of drug use is currently being discussed at several levels, and the Government is considering a revision of the Criminal Code.

Surveillance Needs and Additional Studies

Trust points are available through several outlets, and HIV cases identified in these outlets are reported to a national database. Health behavioral surveys have also been conducted in the country, and the Government is eager to improve its overall health database. For example, the Government is currently working on the development of a birth registry, since infant and maternal mortality data are currently not a reliable source of information for health planning and assessment. UNAIDS, together with United Nations Development Program (UNDP), has carried out studies of seroprevalence and rapid response assessments. NGOs carry out sociological and behavioral surveys of highly vulnerable groups such as IDUs and CSWs. However, Government officials consider that to get a clearer picture of health sector issues, data are also necessary in several other areas: 1) on adolescents aged 15 to18 years; 2) on IDUs regarding HIV/AIDS risk behavior; 3) on risk behaviors and seroprevalence in prisons; 3) on over-prescription of antibiotics by physicians; 4) on training needs for the rational use of drugs; and 5) on resistance to antibiotics for STIs. With support from USAID, CDC has initiated training of MoH staff on sentinel surveillance.

Vulnerable and Highly Vulnerable Groups

The Kyrgyz Republic is actively promoting needle-exchange programs, which according to evidence shown in other countries, significantly reduces the spread of infectious disease among IDUs. Currently, 1,400 IDUs have access to free syringes in Bishkek, Takmak, and Osh. On average, the programs register a 90 percent rate of needle return. Innovative approaches have been used to tackle the STI epidemic such as provision of information and care to CSWs, introduction of the WHO-recommended public health approach to STI prevention and treatment, including the syndromic approach to STI management, and monitoring STI antimicrobial resistance. Public services and many NGOs work with highly vulnerable groups, such as IDUs, CSWs, and MSM, but these groups are insufficiently covered. UN agencies, bilateral agencies and foundations such as Soros Foundation/OSI provide assistance to national agencies.

The Ministry of Health services involved in prevention and treatment of drug abuse, HIV/AIDS, and STIs, and in ensuring blood safety include the AIDS National Association, five oblast AIDS Prevention centers and 36 laboratories with a staff of about 200, the National Narcology Center, the National Dermatology and Venereal Dispensary, and the National Blood Transfusion Center. The Ministries of Education, Defense, Labor, and Internal Affairs as well as regional and local authorities are also involved in HIV/AIDS prevention. National authorities closely cooperate with numerous national NGOs that cover many areas of drug abuse and HIV/AIDS prevention.

UNICEF (2002) reports that 58 percent of young people aged 14–17 are aware of use of condoms as a means of HIV prevention. Yet despite high levels of awareness, the message is not getting through clearly enough to young people. Teenagers are poorly covered by prevention efforts, and there is a strong need to reach out to those who dropped out or are likely to drop out of school. Peer education and an IEC campaign are needed for vulnerable young people—those who are not necessarily at risk now but who can be at risk in the future. Posters and printed materials need to be prepared with participation of representatives from those groups. Leaders of both the Muslim and the Christian Orthodox communities have been approached and have become supportive of condom use and needle-exchange programs, except in schools.

The Republican Center for Health Promotion advocates intersectoral policies on healthy lifestyles and educational programs in partnership with NGOs, local communities, and schools. Together with the Ministry of Education and WHO, the Center works on health promotion in schools, having started four pilot projects in September 2002 and teaching health subjects in first and fifth grades. About 10 percent of the teachers involved in this program have already been trained. Furthermore, the Center works on raising awareness about HIV/AIDS, and on prevention of drug addiction with the Ministry of Interior. The Union of Educational Institutions of the Kyrgyz Republic is an association that provides consultations, information, coordination, and training on HIV/AIDS to students, parents, and teachers in the entire republic.

The NGO Bely Zhurav focuses on the youth in the army, and has been carrying out an IEC campaign for soldiers on prevention of HIV/AIDS and STIs, and providing legal and medical assistance to those who are HIV infected. According to this NGO, which works with assistance from UNDP, all administrative levels of the Ministry of Defense have understood the importance of prevention work. The NGO will also carry out activities in the Ministry of Interior. There are about 10–12,000 soldiers in the Ministry of Defense and 20–36,000 in the Ministry of Interior. The NGO Biom is a youth ecological movement, which mainly provides education on household ecology, but also has training programs on healthy lifestyle (that partially cover HIV/AIDS and TB prevention) and primary prevention in schools.

Preventive, Diagnostic, and Treatment Issues
Under a new UNDP/UNAIDS program starting next year, methadone will be distributed free to female IDUs and HIV-positive IDUs. Taken orally under medical supervision, methadone reduces the risk of infection from needle sharing. Family doctors are involved in prevention and treatment activities. The Association of Groups of Family Doctors trains family doctors on appropriate treatment of TB, HIV/AIDS and STIs, assisted by the Soros Foundation/OSI and USAID. The Association carries out workshops on proper practices of HIV/AIDS prevention and diagnosis, which will be replicated throughout the Republic. The Association has been working with USAID on a pilot project in Chui, where there is a large number of drug users. No information is available on MTCT in the Kyrgyz Republic.

NGO and Partner Activities
The Kyrgyz Republic has a very strong presence of NGO activities in the country, with over 5,000 NGOs registered. A Council of Public Organizations, which is chaired by the President of the Kyrgyz Republic, includes representatives of NGOs. NGOs involved in the work with IDUs meet once a year. Examples of the work of some of the active NGOs are provided below.

■ Socium is an NGO that works with drug addicts covering Bishkek and Chui Oblast. It provides medical assistance for IDUs; offers behavioral and sociological support; trains outreach workers on harm reduction support; and works on prevention of HIV/AIDS among drug users. Socium is now covering about 4,000 IDUs, while funding is only available for

700 IDUs, and is increasingly covering women. This NGO is a member of the Central European Network on Harm Reduction, and receives part of the condoms distributed from the Republican AIDS Center. The NGO Sanitas Charity Fund deals with drug addiction amongst teenagers, providing treatment.

■ Tais Plus is supported by UNDP to work on HIV/AIDS and STIs prevention for CSWs. This NGO started in 1998 and is now covering more than 80 percent of the country, covering 90 percent of the CSWs in Bishkek, and CSWs in other cities, but only distributes 10 percent of the necessary condoms. The price per condom is about 5 som (12 cents), which many CSWs cannot afford. This NGO is also carrying out an IEC campaign, including training, workshops, information materials and condom promotion; provides free medical services at anonymous centers supported by WHO; and works with law enforcement bodies.

■ Oasis is an NGO that works with men who have sex with men by providing information on the prevention of HIV/AIDS and STIs and legal support for MSM. The NGO has about 5,000 MSM clients. Since homosexuality is usually concealed, it is difficult to reach this group and organize it. MSM are also a diverse social mix, including high-level officials, married men, and poorly educated people in rural areas. Oasis conducts workshops, develops informational materials, and distributes condoms. Condom use among MSM increased from 5 percent in 1997 to 35 percent in 2001. However, more funding is necessary for condoms.

UN agencies, bilateral agencies, and the Soros Foundation/OSI have also been very active in drug use, HIV/AIDS, and STIs prevention in the Kyrgyz Republic. However, it is estimated that only about 2 to 5 percent of drug users are covered by harm reduction programs, at a cost of $30,000/year for 1,000 clients (only for syringes).

A Multi-Sectoral Committee on HIV/AIDS Prevention, supported by UNDP and Soros Foundation/OSI, provides peer education and needle exchange to highly vulnerable groups through a network of 25 NGOs spread throughout the country. The Committee has also prepared educational programs on healthy lifestyles. UNDP has contributed $800,000 for HIV/AIDS prevention and treatment since 1997, having assisted the government to set up the National Program, and has now a $510,000 program for the next five years.

The Soros Foundation/OSI has been working since 1999 with UNDP on prevention programs, which are now partially funded by $110,000 from USAID. The first pilot projects for 700 drug users were implemented in Bishkek and Osh. In Bishkek drug users are more open (attend psychotherapy sessions on how to prevent overdose, how to prepare drugs in a safe way, etc.). Soros Foundation/OSI has also followed up on a needle exchange program for CSWs that was initially established by the AIDS Foundation East West (a spin-off of MSF). Although OSI works with the Ministry of Interior, some officials are against HR as they fear that it promotes use of drugs. A prison program includes education and distribution of bleach, but not needle exchange. Soros Foundation/OSI has also started a pilot methadone program for 50 clients, but which has been providing treatment to only 28 clients, of which eight are HIV positive. This program costs $3,000 per yr for 100 people. The Ministry of Justice is expected to allow the establishment of a methadone program in prisons. Soros Foundation/OSI also works with street children, using cartoons to educate children about drug abuse and HIV/AIDS, as suggested by Street Kids International (a Canadian NGO). The Ministry of Education has not yet included education on drug abuse and HIV/AIDS in the school curriculum. Thus this program is only carried out through local NGOs.

UNICEF has been chairing the UN-Theme Group, and has been carrying out a four-year program for 2000–2004 with US$4 million that includes HIV/AIDS activities. UNICEF carried out a Knowledge, attitudes and practices (KAP) baseline study in five oblasts (Narine, Osh, Chio, Issy-kul, Babken), assessing the knowledge of 15 to18-years-old on sexual behavior, STIs, and

HIV/AIDS. It works on a health promotion program with the Ministries of Health and Education, and five radio stations. The health promotion program focuses on HIV prevention and healthy life skills and attitudes; and involves peer education to strengthen youth organizations, making sure services for youth are friendly and accessible (involve youth in design). The Youth Program is now being scaled up, aiming at having at least one hour per week of healthy life skills taught in schools. UNICEF is also assisting NGOs in working with street children to raise funding and establish shelters.

UNFPA works with the National AIDS Center addressing heterosexual transmission, which is estimated to be responsible for more than 20 percent of the HIV positive cases. STIs among university students are increasing rapidly (as many female students would be involved in occasional sex for money). UNFPA is also working with UNICEF in schools and training school teachers; and with the IPPF and Association for Reproductive Health (NGO), which carried out a study on awareness and knowledge about reproductive health. Condom availability is uneven, and UNFPA is unable to cover all the needs. In 2002, DFID and the Government of Netherlands covered 80 percent of the condom needs for highly vulnerable groups, and the local government in Osh allocated $24,000 for condom procurement. The religious community poses some obstacles to this work. Although the religious community has made commitments to reproductive health rights and to prevention of HIV/AIDS, it opposes discussions on safe sex and the distribution of condoms in schools. UNFPA organized a roundtable with religious leaders, and it was expecting their endorsement of the Law on Reproductive Rights.

The UN High Commission on Refugees (UNHCR) focuses on reproductive health and HIV/AIDS among refugee youth, who mostly come from Tajikistan (but are ethnically Kyrgyz), but also include Chechens and Afghans. UNHCR supports NGO-based awareness campaigns among refugee youth, condoms distribution, and clinics for refugees. The International Organization for Migration (IOM) works on a public information campaign for labor migrants. Labor migrants usually lack access to health care and are more vulnerable to HIV/AIDS. Many women end up in forced sex labor or resort to CSW as a temporary way to earn income until they get regular jobs. In Kyrgyz, blood tests are required for official work, and therefore, ethnic Kyrgyz returning from Tajikistan, Uzbekistan, and other countries, have to pass an HIV test to become citizens.

USAID has been assisting HIV/AIDS prevention activities in Kyrgyz in the context of the implementation of its Central Asia Strategy, which includes $2 million for prevention programs over the next two years. USAID has also been supporting US CDC activities, including training the Ministry of Health staff in sentinel surveillance. DFID allocated an initial $2 million for HR programs, and is providing support to restructure the penal system. The Swiss Cooperation Office has provided 160,000 Swiss francs to an information program on drug use in Osh, targeting students and training teachers. It opened the Rainbow Information Center, which provides support to the program in Jalal-Abad and Batken Oblasts.

Donors and NGOs have referred the need to scale up HR programs to cover 60 percent of highly vulnerable groups (IDUs, CSWs), and ensure the long-term sustainability of HIV/AIDS prevention and treatment activities in the Kyrgyz Republic; providing school drop outs with information and education on HIV/AIDS; dealing with the issue of stigma; decriminalizing drug use; reducing overcrowding in prisons; and supporting expanded methadone substitution treatment for IDUs.

Funding

The Kyrgyz Republic allocated 1.8 percent of the GDP to the health sector in 2000 (12 percent of total public expenditures), which resulted in less than $7 per capita on health. The Government stated that in 2001 it allocated about $1 million for the implementation of the second HIV/AIDS program, but the first HIV/AIDS Program only obtained 18 percent of the planned funding, and thus disbursement for the second program is worth attention. The Joint Program with UNDP and UNAIDS had $250,000 funding. HR programs are supported by UN agencies,

Soros Foundation/OSI, and the local government in Osh. The GFATM approved a $5 million grant for HIV/AIDS out of a request of $17 million that had been prepared with assistance from UNAIDS. This will complement expected funding from public and other sources (of about $5 million) for 2003–2007.

Tuberculosis Epidemiological Profile

The Kyrgyz Republic is second among Central Asian Republics in the incidence of TB. The 30-year downward trend in TB incidence in the Kyrgyz Republic, as in the rest of the FSU, was reversed in the early 1990s (Table 16). From 1990 to 1999, yearly incidence increased in the Kyrgyz Republic from 53/100,000 population to 132. An incidence rate of 10/100,000 is considered by WHO to be of critical significance. There are over 6,000 new cases of TB annually and about 7,000 prevalent "chronic" TB cases. In 1996, a pilot DOTS program was established in four districts of two regions of the country. After encouraging results from the use of new approaches in new cases of TB (treatment success rate of 88 percent in 1996 and case finding higher by 14 percent than in the rest of the country), DOTS was introduced in the entire country in 1998. This expansion was orchestrated through the health reform program undertaken by the Kyrgyz Ministry of Health and supported by a World Bank credit. More than one third of the primary health care budget of this credit has been allocated to TB training, diagnosis, and treatment. Introduction of DOTS did lead to an immediate improvement in the epidemiological situation in Kyrgyz Republic. Partly as a result of better detection efforts, TB reporting and mortality rates continued to grow significantly till 1999. In 2000, for the first time since 1993, TB reporting decreased. However, it is too early to judge whether the tide of the epidemic is reversed.

TABLE 16. TUBERCULOSIS RATES, KYRGYZ (PER 100,000 CIVILIAN POPULATION)	1990	1995	2000	2001
TB death rate	7.2	13.4	12.6	13.5
TB prevalence rate	228.5	246.1	363.8	313
% of newly notified cases with BK+	31	25	22	24
TB case notification	2,306	3,266	5,953	6,274
TB case notification rate	53	72.4	121.8	127.3
-among males	59.3	90.1	145.3	146.9
-among females	44.9	55.1	97.9	107.2
-among children	20.2	28.3	57.5	77

Source: National TB Institute.

At the end of 2001, there were 15,420 registered patients with active TB disease—a more than 50 percent increase since 1990. Between 1990 and 2001, the notification rate increased almost 3 times, and the death rate increased by almost twice. Although the TB notification rate of 127/100,000 of population is the second highest in the WHO European region, which includes Central Asia, the WHO Global TB control surveillance program estimates that only 82 percent of all new TB cases were reported in 2000. Since 1999, however, the growth rate of the TB epidemic has slowed down to 5 percent a year compared to 17 percent between 1995 and 1998. The TB death rate has slightly improved from 16/100,000 in 1997 to 12.6 in 2000, but in 2002 returned to the 1999 level of 13.6.

TB case notification varies significantly across the country. The highest rate of almost 150/100,000 was reported in Jalal Abad in the South of the country, as compared to the country average of 127, while the lowest rates are around 70. There are records of districts with reporting rates of over 200. One of the reasons for the increase in TB rates among the civilian population in 2001 was the release of 1,603 prisoners with active TB.

The TB situation in prisons is alarming (Table 17). In 2001, the reporting rate of new TB cases was over 60 times that in the civilian population, and the death rate was almost 200 times higher. At the end of 2001, there were 2,188 TB cases in prisons, from which 686 died. Although the prison population accounts for just about 0.5 percent of the total population, in 2000 and 2001 nearly as much or even more TB deaths occurred in prisons than in the civilian population. In 2001, one out of three inmates with active TB died. Between 1995 and 2001, the TB reporting rate in prisons increased more than nine times, and the TB death rate increased more than ten times.

TABLE 17. TB in Prisons in the Kyrgyz Republic

	1990	1995	2000	2001
Prison inmates with active	–	–	2,580	2,188
Prisons inmates newly detected with TB	–	174	1,422	1,992
Prisons inmates who died of TB	–	56	542	686
TB death rate (per 100,000)	–	262.2	1887.4	2635.9
Prison TB facilities	1	1	3	3

Sources of information: Ministry of Interior.

The TB epidemiological situation in prisons contributes to the growth of mortality due to TB. There is a wide agreement in the Kyrgyz Government that the number of prisoners is too high; compounding this burden is the fact that the prison sector has not adopted the DOTS strategy, and TB patients in prisons remain virtually incurable due to lack of financing. There is no effective mechanism of referral of TB patients from prison to TB Dispensaries.

Strategies, Policies, and Legal Framework

Government commitment is high, as demonstrated by the adoption of the two consecutive National Tuberculosis Control Programs (NTP). National interagency meetings on TB, and more recently on TB and HIV/AIDS, have been held annually, and have been chaired by the President of the Kyrgyz Republic, Prime Minister, and Deputy Prime Minister. The Law on TB prevention was adopted in 1998. The Government has been considering several additional measures that could have a positive impact on TB control: decriminalization of drug use to decrease overcrowding in prisons; decreasing time spent in prison before sentence; and not permitting amnesty for prisoners with TB. The Government is, however, planning to implement a DOTS Plus program for diagnosis and treatment of multi-drug resistant TB, which is a cause of concern for NGOs and donors.

The number of prisoners (20,000) is high for the size of the population, but it is in the middle range among FSU countries. The Ministry of Justice (MOJ) aims at reducing the numbers of prisoners by about 1,200–1,300 per year. This will be accomplished by introducing alternative forms of punishment, moving to shorter sentences, focusing on preventing factors leading to repeated offenses, and addressing underlying factors behind crime and development of criminal careers. The Kyrgyz system of prisons has been administratively under the Ministry of Internal Affairs (MOIA), but actions have been undertaken by the Kyrgyz Government to move these institutions to the MOJ. The MOJ has launched a wide set of preparatory measures aimed at introducing fundamental penal system changes (Kokko 2002). What is also needed is a consistent treatment strategy to assure that prisoners released with TB have someplace to be treated and to receive social support.

Surveillance Needs and Additional Studies

Surveillance is based on quarterly cohort analysis according to WHO standard definitions. There is no systematic surveillance of MDRTB, but available data suggest that MDRTB is high (7 percent among new cases and 37 percent among previously treated cases), (Table 18). Drug resistance surveillance is not linked with TB notification and is limited to some geographical areas (cases diagnosed at the National Reference Laboratory and drug susceptibility testing—DST—done on selected cases). Funded by USAID, CDC provided laboratory training at the National TB Research Institute.

TABLE 18. REPORTED TB CASES, KYRGYZ REPUBLIC							
	New		Previously treated		Unknown		Total
	N	%	N	%	N	%	N
Tested	141	100	81	100	96	100	318
Resistant to INH	33	23.4	43	53.1	39	40.6	115
Resistant to RMP	18	12.8	36	44.4	24	25.0	78
Multidrug resistant §	9	6.4	30	37.0	20	20.8	59

* Drug susceptibility testing; ß resistant to at least INH and RMP

Source: Euro TB (2002). InVS/KNCV. Surveillance of tuberculosis in Europe.

Preventive, Diagnostic, and Treatment Issues

In 1996, the Kyrgyz Republic, with assistance from the WHO and the World Bank, was first among the Central Asian countries to start implementation of DOTS. The National TB Program for 1996–2000 (NTP-I) was approved by a Government Resolution in 1995. Priority was given to detection of infectious (smear sputum positive) TB cases by sputum microscopy among self-reporting symptomatic TB cases; standardized short course chemotherapy regimens with reliable drug supply; monitoring and evaluation system based on standard international definitions; and quarterly cohort analysis of treatment outcomes. The revised NTP-II is closely related with the World Bank health reform project objectives, aimed at providing:

- Enhanced primary health care network allowing integration of TB services and better access to TB diagnosis and treatment.
- Rational utilization of inpatient care resulting from wider application of ambulatory treatment for TB.
- Health care provider payment improvement allowing staff incentives for quality TB case management.
- Improved pharmaceutical management allowing ensured supply of TB drugs.

The Kyrgyz Republic had inherited the Soviet TB control strategy based on active detection of respiratory TB cases via regular (once in 6–24 months) mass X-ray screening (MMR) of the population, and lengthy (8–12 months) individualized treatment regimens administered almost exclusively on an inpatient basis in TB facilities (Table 19). The evaluation of treatment effectiveness was conducted through an annual (vs. quarterly cohort) analysis.

Presently, TB detection is based on sputum microscopy and X-ray screening of population groups with high risk of TB. Both detection and diagnosis are made at primary health care facilities, including family group practices. Hospitalization in TB facilities is limited to two months of intensive treatment or is fully administered on an ambulatory basis by the primary health care network. The average length of stay was reduced between 1995 and 2001 from 101 inpatient days per patient treated to 74. Monitoring of treatment is based on sputum examinations at set intervals using international standardized treatment outcome definitions.

As a result of the NTP-I implementation, population coverage by DOTS expanded from 5 percent in 1996–1997 to 100 percent by 1999. The WHO target of 85 percent for TB treatment success rate was achieved among new civilian TB cases registered for treatment in 1999 and 2000. Average length of stay in TB hospitals was reduced from 101 inpatient days per patient treated to 74 days per patient between 1995 and 2001. However, the NTP has not yet been entirely successful. This could be explained in part by lack of financing of the health sector. The epidemic situation continues to worsen although at a lower rate than before 2000. Stagnation or even increase in TB mortality in 2001 is worrisome. The high treatment success rate at the onset of the DOTS introduction (88 percent in 1996) was followed by a drop to 76 percent in 1997 and was below the WHO target of 85 percent in 1998–99 patient cohorts (82 and 83 percent, respectively). There is no decrease in mortality rates, which did, in fact, increase by about 1 percent in 1999 and 7 percent in 2001.

No TB drugs are produced domestically. All TB drugs for new TB cases are procured in a centralized fashion by the MOH with funding from the World Bank and KfW. TB drugs procured by the MOH are free of charge to TB patients, regardless of their place of residence.

TABLE 19. TB Services in the Kyrgyz Republic

	1990	1995	2000	2001
TB facilities	74	77	77	75
TB sanatoria	9	–	–	–
TB offices in general health care facilities	41	41	35	34
TB beds	5,900	4,185	3,770	3,374
- in TB sanatoria	2,090	–	–	–
- in general health care facilities	3,810	4,185	3,770	3,374
TB physicians	334	313	314	308
- in specialist TB sanatoria	67	–	–	–
- in general health care facilities	334	313	314	308
Nurses providing TB care	708	512	464	408
Sanitary nurses providing TB care	714	471	429	373
Inpatient days	701,442	811,664	1,180,726	1,167,363
- in TB sanatoria	432,432	–	–	–
- in general health care facilities	269,010	811,664	1,180,726	1,167,363
Average length of stay in TB facilities	91	101	76	74
Outpatient visits by TB patients	480,100	515,421	522,634	463,165
Surgeries in TB patients	162	183	218	271
Radiography tests made to TB patients	1,132,100	40,987	41,526	52,225
Radiography machines	559	551	548	504
Fluorography machines	93	97	111	101
Screening radiography tests (MMR)	2,274,300	647,841	715,751	693,891
% of people who underwent screening radiography tests	52	14	15	14
BCG vaccinations and revaccinations	117,780	109,217	89,492	90,103
BCG Revaccinations	2484	1073	103	105
Sputum smears for detection of TB		59,891	61,726	77,821
Sputum culture tests	9,465	7,324	8,436	8,926
Sputum DST (drug susceptibility tests) for TB	711	541	961	620

Source: Ministry of Health.

NGO and Partner Activities

The Association of Groups of Family Doctors trains family doctors on proper methods of diagnosis and treatment of TB, as well as prevention and treatment of HIV/AIDS, and STIs. The Association has obtained a grant from the Soros Foundation/OSI to replicate the program throughout the Republic. Numerous other NGOs operate in Kyrgyz Republic, and Table 20 summarizes the activity of the main international partners.

TABLE 20. PARTNER ACTIVITIES ON TB, KYRGYZ REPUBLIC			
Implementing Agency	Funding Agency	Coverage	Area of Activity
CDC	USAID	Nationwide	▪ Quality assurance of TB laboratories in the Central TB Laboratory and regional TB laboratories; ▪ Laboratory training
HOPE	USAID	Nationwide	▪ DOTS training of TB specialists and primary health care physicians all over the country (71 TB specialists, general health care practitioners (FGP) and epidemiologists since July 2001); ▪ Provision of TB drugs and lab equipment (Biological Safety Cabinet) ▪ Lab quality control ▪ DOTS program monitoring
MoH	KfW		▪ Since 1997 to 2005: DM 10 million for first line TB drugs, lab equipment and supplies

Funding

The Kyrgyz Government has very limited funding for TB overall and is heavily reliant on the donor community. DOTS have not yet implemented in prisons due to lack of financing. However, the allocation for the NTP from the national budget increased from 21.5 million soms (US$434,300) in 1996 to 64.6 million soms (US$1,3 million) in 2000. In 1997, the Government also obtained a US$1.6 million credit from the World Bank, as part of the Health Reform Project, and in 1996–2005, a total of DM10 million from KfW for DOTS implementation. The Country Coordination Mechanism has obtained $1.2 million from the GFATM for DOTS and DOTS Plus implementation. This will add to approximately $11 million expected from public and other sources for the period 2003–2007.

In 1997, the Government obtained support from KfW in the amount of DM5million for first line TB drugs, and lab and X-ray equipment. USAID, through its implementing partners (Project HOPE and CDC), provided $70,000 to equip the National Reference TB laboratory and $42,000 for DOTS training at the National TB Research Institute. The Soros Foundation/OSI provided $59,000 for TB drugs, training, and equipment. The DOTS strategy was introduced in the entire country in 1998. This expansion was orchestrated through the health reform program undertaken by the Kyrgyz Ministry of Health and supported by a World Bank credit. More than one-third of the primary health care budget of this loan has been allocated to TB training, diagnosis, and treatment. Of the total amount of US$8.5 million for four years, US$1.6 million was for implementation of DOTS-based TB control, with coverage to grow from 22 to 55 rayons (financing TB drugs, lab and X-ray equipment, and program monitoring).

Additional funding is necessary to assure an uninterrupted supply of drugs and supplies, as well as lab and X-ray equipment, and DOTS training for the MOH and prisons. In addition, funds are also needed for a drug resistance prevalence survey; community mobilization (including NGOs) and public education; publication of training and educational materials; training of prison health staff on DOTS; and food for TB patients, particularly in prisons.

CHAPTER 6

COUNTRY PROFILE: TAJIKISTAN

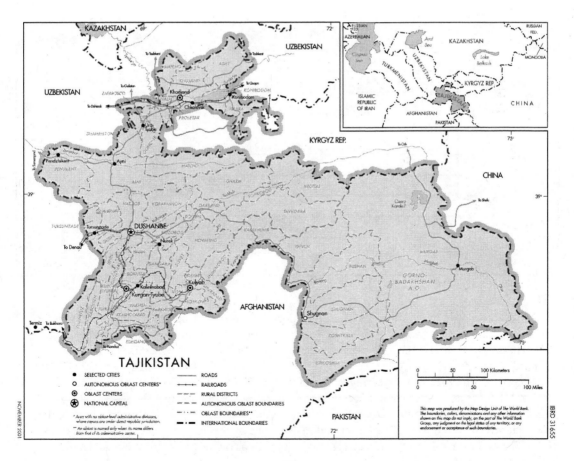

TAJIKISTAN

- ● SELECTED CITIES
- ○ AUTONOMOUS OBLAST CENTERS*
- ◉ OBLAST CENTERS
- ✪ NATIONAL CAPITAL

- ﹉﹉﹉ ROADS
- ┼┼┼┼ RAILROADS
- ﹉ ﹉ RURAL DISTRICTS
- ﹏﹏﹏ AUTONOMOUS OBLAST BOUNDARIES
- ﹏ · ﹏ OBLAST BOUNDARIES**
- ▬ · ▬ INTERNATIONAL BOUNDARIES

* Areas with no oblast-level administrative divisions, where rayons are under direct republic jurisdiction.

** An oblast is named only when its name differs from that of its administrative center.

NOVEMBER 2001

This map was produced by the Map Design Unit of The World Bank. The boundaries, colors, denominations and any other information shown on this map do not imply, on the part of The World Bank Group, any judgment on the legal status of any territory, or any endorsement or acceptance of such boundaries.

IBRD 31655

ajikistan is the poorest ECA country, with an annual per capita income of $170. According to official data, 80 percent of the population live in poverty, and according to Bank estimates, 30 percent may be unemployed. As reported by Central Asia News, between 30 to 50 percent of Tajikistan's economic activity is linked to narcotics trafficking, and the number of Tajiks using hard drugs such as opium and heroin, has been steeply increasing. Tajikistan's economic dependency on drug trafficking creates many barriers against containing the pending drug-related epidemic of HIV/AIDS. Some foreign experts in Tajikistan assert that the elimination of trafficking-related economic activity would have a serious impact on living standards in an already very poor country. The breakdown of the Soviet Union was also followed by a civil war that disrupted the lives of many people, and the normal functioning of health services, and led to increased migration. All of these factors can support the growth of the HIV/AIDS epidemic.

HIV/AIDS Epidemiological Profile

According to official statistics, Tajikistan had only 92 HIV-infected persons and 1 person with AIDS in April 2003, but two thirds of the cases were reported in 2001 and 2002. Among those infected, 65 percent are IDUs, but 19 percent are of unknown cause. According to survey data reported by national and UNAIDS experts, the actual number of HIV infected may be 10 times higher. In some regions, this figure could be 20 times higher or more, but limited laboratory services do not allow collection of sentinel surveillance data from vulnerable groups. As in other Central Asian countries, the growth of the epidemic since first established in 1995 has been significant (Table 21), and it is mainly concentrated on male (56 percent) IDUs.

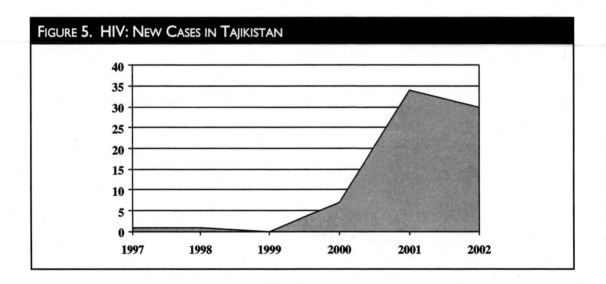

FIGURE 5. HIV: NEW CASES IN TAJIKISTAN

Intravenous drug use with needle sharing is the predominant mode of transmission. Over 6,000 drug addicts are officially registered, but the Government estimates that the number of IDUs is 30,000, and UNODCCP estimates that the real number of drug users is closer to 100,000. About 4,500 drug users were registered in Dushanbe alone, and many of these (93 percent) report sharing needles and syringes; therefore the AIDS Center expects the number of cases of HIV infected IDUs to rise steeply in the capital in the near future. A substantial part of Tajikistan's economic activity is unofficially linked to drug trafficking. In 2001, law enforcement officials intercepted 8.8 tons of drugs, including 4.2 tons of heroin, a 26 percent increase over 2000. The quantities of raw poppy seeds seized indicates also that heroin production laboratories now exist in the country.

There are an estimated 5,000 of CSW, 500 of whom are based in Dushanbe. The average age of CSWs is 20–25 years, but very young girls, 12–13-year-olds, are also involved in CSW. An official assessment showed that 20 percent of CSW inject drugs and provide sexual services in exchange for money to buy the drugs. CSWs do not have adequate access to condoms, and clients of low-paid CSWs usually do not use condoms. Therefore, it is not surprising that, since 1993, the number of sexually transmitted infections has been increasing, especially in this vulnerable group. The incidence of syphilis in 2001 is eight times higher than in 1991. In Dushanbe, during the period 1993–2000, syphilis incidence was 3–6 times higher than for the country as a whole. About 40 percent of registered cases of STIs are among married women, according to official statistics, indicating substantial extramarital sexual contact among their partners. However, these data underestimate the impact of STIs, since there is incomplete notification of cases due to the fact that very few patients use public treatment services for STI.

TABLE 21. NEWLY-DIAGNOSED HIV INFECTIONS, TAJIKISTAN

	Up to 1995	1996	1997	1998	1999	2000	2001	2002	Total
Tajikistan	2	–	1	1	–	7	34	30	92

Source: AIDS Center, Ministry of Health. Total refers to April 2003

Strategies, Policies, and Legal Framework

With assistance from the UNAIDS Theme Group, the Government of Tajikistan prepared a Strategic Plan for the period 2002–2005 to control HIV/AIDS in the Republic of Tajikistan. Despite the low level of HIV infection (according to official statistics), and the enormous pressure placed on a crumbling health care system by transition and civil war, the political leadership has demonstrated strong commitment to HIV/AIDS prevention. The first cases of HIV were detected in 1991. In 1991, the Center on HIV/AIDS Control was established and branches set up in the oblasts. In 1993, a Law was adopted on HIV/AIDS Control and a new version of that law is currently being drafted. A Government Resolution in 1997 established the National Coordination Committee for HIV/AIDS Prevention, which is headed by the Deputy Prime Minister of the Republic of Tajikistan. The 1st National Program was adopted in 1997 and a 2nd National Program up to 2007 was adopted on December 30, 2000. These actions highlight the country's proactive approach in securing an expanded response to the HIV/AIDS threat.

The National Program outlines the key policy directions, strategies, and priority interventions for HIV/AIDS and STIs. The National Program policy is founded on the following elements:

- HIV/AIDS and STIs are problems that affect the whole society and call for political and financial support from the Government;
- There is a need for a multi-sectoral approach that involves ministries, NGOs, and donor agencies;
- Information about HIV/AIDS status should be kept confidential and disclosed only to the persons tested and those referred to in the Law on AIDS Prevention;
- It is essential to integrate the prevention and care dimensions into the programs and actions on HIV/AIDS and STI prevention and control, blood transfusion, family planning, and mother and child health programs;
- The National coordinating mechanism for the National Program implementation was established in 1997 and extended in 2002;
- Care for and protection of HIV-infected people should be secured;

▨ Issues of condom promotion and distribution, as well as provision of medicines for HIV/AIDS and STI patients should be addressed;

▨ Wide dissemination of information about HIV/AIDS and STIs among the population, particularly among youth and risk groups, is essential.

Surveillance Needs and Additional Studies

Because of absence of confirmatory tests for HIV diagnosis (immunoblot method), primary HIV-positive blood samples are being tested in laboratories located in Kazakhstan and the Russian Federation. However, no sentinel surveillance has been conducted among highly vulnerable groups, and screening to assure blood safety is deficient. The AIDS Center has carried out studies twice amongst IDUs and only 1 to 2 HIV cases have been found. This is probably because of the low quality of tests and the fact that testing was done on a voluntary basis. However, CDC has recently initiated activities in the country, and under the GFATM grant, investments on upgrading the lab network were planned.

Vulnerable and Highly Vulnerable Groups

AIDS Centers have been established in Dushanbe and all regional centers. These Centers coordinate HIV/AIDS prevention activities of dispensaries for STIs and TB, narcology centers, and blood transfusion units. AIDS Centers promote the work of NGOs with vulnerable groups. With the support of UNAIDS, international NGOs (Soros Foundation/OSI, USAID), and local municipalities, 15 Trust Points for IDUs and one pilot project for CSWs were established to work with vulnerable and highly vulnerable groups. Specialists working in these settings (a drug abuse specialist, a psychotherapist, a STI physician) render consultations, exchange used syringes and needles, provide condoms, and disseminate educational materials. Former drug users work as volunteers. However, the AIDS Center estimates that only about 5 percent of IDUs in the country, and 10 percent of IDUs in Dushanbe, are being covered by preventive activities. Under the GFATM grant, the CCM plans to open 13 additional Trust Points to cover 40 percent of IDUs in the country. Prevention of HIV/AIDS among drug addicts is not considered by law enforcement agencies as a priority. No services for drug addicts exist in the country.

Condom availability in the country is poor, and the majority of IDUs and CSWs cannot afford to buy condoms. All condoms available in the market are sold through drug stores. Storage rules are not observed, and vendors do not possess information about the specifications, date of production, and expiration date of condoms.

The UNAIDS rapid assessment showed that 60 percent of the population are not aware of HIV/AIDS infection routes and prevention measures, especially in rural areas, where 70 percent of the population lives. According to UNICEF (2000), only 24 percent of young people aged 14–17 are aware of the need to use condoms as a means of preventing HIV infection, the lowest rate in the region. Among women aged 30–49, approximately 10 percent are aware of the need to use condoms to prevent infection, while only 7 percent of the younger group of women (aged 15–29 years) is aware of this prevention measure. The HIV/AIDS Program includes an educational campaign for youth and adults, and it has published textbooks about HIV/AIDS infection for use in schools.

Preventive, Diagnostic, and Treatment Issues

Only STI dispensaries and a private center ("Zoukhra," in Dushanbe) have the legal right to diagnose and treat STIs. Officially, diagnosis and treatment are free of charge. In reality, the patient must pay for most of these medical services, and he or she has to cover the cost of pharmaceuticals. Patients can also receive free hospital treatment, but in that case their personal data would be reported, which makes treatment undesirable for vulnerable group members who fear being exposed.

NGO and Partner Activities

The UN-Theme Group is very active and well organized in Tajikistan, including co-sponsors of UNAIDS, international NGOs, and bilateral agencies. It operates in close collaboration with national experts and local NGOs. Although the main focus of the work is on youth, it has been contentious to address HIV/AIDS and STIs prevention in school programs. A manual for trainers on how to teach and explain HIV/AIDS and a new textbook on "Healthy Lifestyles" for teachers of the secondary schools were developed. These cover various issues such as drug use, reproductive health, HIV/AIDS, STIs, and tobacco. The Ministry of Education selected 60 pilot schools where trained teachers will start educating students on healthy lifestyles.

Funding

While the goals of the HIV, AIDS, and STIs control programs are well articulated, the Government faces serious constraints in funding health care in general. The Government provides some funding for the HIV/AIDS National Program from the national budget, mainly for infrastructure and labs, but most of the assistance has been provided by member organizations of the UN-Theme Group on AIDS, including UNFPA, UNDP, UNICEF, Soros Foundation/OSI, and other organizations. The Ministry of Health provided a more accessible facility to house the AIDS Center, which still needs rehabilitation. The GFATM awarded a grant of $600,000 for HIV/AIDS prevention for the period 2003 to 2004, and the Bank may award an IDA credit on HIV/AIDS in 2005. UNICEF has been implementing a four year program (2000–2004) of $6 million that includes HIV/AIDS prevention activities with youth. However, additional funding is necessary to improve the health infrastructure, labs, blood safety, and work with other vulnerable groups.

Tuberculosis Epidemiological Profile

The TB incidence rate varies between 75/100,000 population and 100, depending on the region, and mortality rates are not as high in Tajikistan as they are in other Central Asian countries, although this may be due to under-reporting. Incidence of TB is higher in large cities. These cities may have more functional TB services, which probably account for better reporting of new cases. However, official data should be treated with caution as they have not been evaluated, and case definitions used are not standardized. The worsening economic and health conditions, poor nutrition, civil war, isolation, and shortage of TB drugs may have all contributed to increased TB incidence in the last 10 years.

TABLE 22. TUBERCULOSIS IN TAJIKISTAN

Year	1995	1996	1997	1998	1999	2000	2001 (11 m.)
Pulmonary smear (new & re-treatment)		232	373	435	622	434	864
Pulmonary smear – TB				1,636	1,589	1,918	1,210
Extra-Pulmonary TB				376	341	427	215
Case notification	1,659	1,647	2,007	2,447	2,552	2,779	2,289
Case notification rate	29	28	31	41	42	46	40
Estimated new cases	4,071	4,557	5,103	5,714	6,395	7,151	7,990
Estimated incidence	71	78	86	95	105	115	127
TB disease detection rate (%)	41	36	39	43	40	39	31
TB mortality rate	N/A	3.0	6.1	N/A	5.9	7.1	N/A

Source: WHO (2002). The 3rd mission on DOTS implementation in Tajikistan.

Official data show rapid decline in TB rates in the early 1990s, which was probably due to the deterioration of case finding (reporting artifact). Even so, between 1993 and 2000, the reported incidence increased four-fold, from 12 to 45 per 100,000 of population. Total TB cases were 2,552 in 1999 and 2,779 in 2000. The WHO estimates are two and half times higher than official reports (6,395 and 7,151, respectively; Table 22). However, the Ministry of Health agrees with WHO experts that the real incidence of TB in Tajikistan may be 3 to 4 times higher than official data indicate. According to the official statistics, the mortality rate among civilians increased by 7 percent between 1999 and 2000, from 6/100,000 to 7. No data are available on the TB situation in prisons to date.

TB is particularly common in the south of the country; the estimated incidence rates over the last few years are well above 100/100,000. According to anecdotal reports, entire villages are affected with TB, and entire families have died of TB. Reported new TB cases decreased approximately 10 percent in 2001, as compared with the previous year. However, active case detection performed in 2001 in a Dushanbe prison, with the help of the NGO Global Partner, has contributed to the total increase in smear positive TB case reporting. TB incidence in children is high; currently there are 45 children under treatment for TB, of which 35 were newly identified in 2001. Again, this should be interpreted with caution, as the lack of any reported fatal cases suggests that misdiagnosis may be common in these patients.

Strategies, Policies and Legal Framework

The Ministry of Health's commitment to implementation of the DOTS strategy is high, and a Five Year National TB Program has been prepared. The Ministry of Health planned to start the program on July 1, 2002, but the Government has not yet fully funded the program. For 2002–2003, a working plan of action deriving from World AIDS Day in Tajikistan has been developed. "Live and let live" is the slogan of the two-year campaign, which will focus on eliminating stigma and discrimination.

Surveillance Needs and Additional Studies

The old Soviet-style notification system continues to be used in Tajikistan. Notification is done on a monthly basis from districts to regions, and on quarterly basis from regions to the National TB Center. Registration forms and registers as recommended by WHO have been prepared in Russian for training purposes, but were not yet printed with the official Ministry of Health logo; therefore, these forms were not yet used.

TABLE 23. TB REPORTING RATE IN TAJIK OBLASTS

Oblast	Location	Notification rate
Dushanbe	Dushanbe	87.3
Dushanbe	Kylyab	75.0
Leninabad	Khujand	N/A
Gorny Badakhshon	Khorugh	N/A
Khatlon	Kurgan Tyube	90.3
Total	Tajikistan	41.8

Source: Ministry of Health 1999.

Preventive, Diagnostic, and Treatment Issues

As with Central Asian countries, Tajikistan inherited the Soviet style TB control strategy, including mass X-ray screening (MMR) and long-term hospitalization for diagnosed cases. However, economic devastation and civil war have made this strategy unaffordable and impossible to pursue. The National TB control program for 1996–2000 failed due to inadequate funding and use of ineffective TB practices. WHO/USAID planned to start support for DOTS implementation in Tajikistan, but the civil war prevented program implementation.

With WHO assistance, however, the Ministry of Health developed the new National TB control program for 2000–2005, which supports adherence to the DOTS strategy and has been endorsed by the Tajik Government. Case finding is officially based on systematic smear examination as the first diagnostic step for symptomatic patients. The NTP adopted the WHO protocol calling for X-ray and fluorography only if three smear examinations are negative and if 10 days of treatment with non-TB specific antibiotics do not result in clinical improvement. The program continues, however, to use expensive and ineffective MMR for TB screening. The military, Ministry of Internal Affairs staff, and prison inmates are expected to undergo compulsory X-ray examinations twice a year. Food sector workers, social workers, sales sector workers, and public education workers are expected to have X-ray examinations once a year. Health workers, army draftees, and World War II veterans are expected to have annual X-ray examinations free of charge. Therefore, over reliance on X-ray diagnosis and over-diagnosis of smear negative cases is common. Systematic and careful monitoring will be necessary to change habits of extensive overuse of X-rays. Application for pension benefits based on X-ray examination should be changed according to the NTP guidelines and replaced by proof of positive smear exam only.

In 2001, WHO, together with Project HOPE, conducted an assessment of the TB situation in Tajikistan, as a preparation for the planned donation of TB drugs by the WHO Global Drug Facility (GDF). As an outcome of this assessment, USAID/CAR decided to support two pilot sites for DOTS implementation, reaching 562,000 people in Dushanbe and 268,000 people in the Leninskiy Rayon (10 km from Dushanbe), representing 13 percent of the country's population. With support from USAID, Project HOPE opened a permanent office in Dushanbe in 2001, and delivered over $70,000 worth of laboratory equipment and reagents. These items will be used to ensure the quality of the laboratory component of the program, a key aspect of DOTS programs. The Ministry of Health adopted standardized TB treatment regimens at the time of the WHO/MSH mission in May 2001, and TB drugs were ordered accordingly through the Global Drug Fund (GDF). However, treatment outcomes provided by the National TB Center for the entire country are not reliable. Standardized regimen in DOTS areas is as follows:

- Category I 2RHZE/4R3H3 (fully supervised)
- Category II 2SRHZE/RHZE/5R3H3E3 (fully supervised)
- Category III 2RHZE/4R3H3 (fully supervised)
- Prophylaxis 6H (without supervision)

The Ministries of Health and Justice agreed in 2001 to start TB treatment in a Dushanbe prison. As mentioned before, active case detection carried out in the prison has contributed to the total increase in smear positive TB case reporting. Out of 421 prisoners screened for TB, about 212 smear positive cases were diagnosed and were treated with a 6-month regimen 2RHZE/4RH. Unfortunately approximately half of the TB cases diagnosed in prison were released, and defaulted after 2 to 3 months of treatment, which led the NGO Global Partner to stop supporting the program.

All TB drugs are imported and are procured by the Ministry of Health centrally via GDF with assistance from Project HOPE. The Indian Government provided TB drugs for 600 patients in 2001. According to anecdotal reports, TB drugs (including Rifampin) are available at pharmacies without prescription, but the prices are prohibitively high relative to incomes. Where DOTS is not available, costs to patients for TB drugs, lab supplies, and X-rays during the course of treatment amount to US$300–400 per patient. Shortages of TB drugs are common, and inappropriate monotherapy continues to be practiced.

The Tajik TB services include the National TB Center in Dushanbe, three regional TB centers, and 5 city and 50 district TB facilities. There are 2,160 beds in 26 functioning TB facilities, but the majority of the facilities require capital renovation. There is a significant shortage of medical equipment: most of the 76 existing X-ray machines are far beyond their useful life and 45 of them are out of order. Only the National TB Center and the three regional TB centers had binocular microscopes in 2000. TB services are staffed by 245 physicians, of which 136 are TB specialists. Many more trained staff will be needed for DOTS expansion.

NGO and Partner Activities

International NGOs including Project HOPE, International Federation of the Red Cross (IFRC), and MERLIN constitute all NGO activity in Tajikistan for TB control (Table 24). WHO and USAID, through Project HOPE and CDC, have been providing active assistance to DOTS in Tajikistan. In addition, the Government of India and NGOs have also provided some assistance, and the Aga Khan Foundation and Global Partner have expressed interest in supporting the program.

Project HOPE has been conducting DOTS training for health staff. Five DOTS medical training courses were held in 2001 in Dushanbe, involving 75 medical staff and 63 nurses coming from Leninsky rayon, Machenton hospital, Dushanbe City Center, and the six Dushanbe polyclinics. Medical staff received a five-day session based on training adapted from the WHO training module on management of TB at district level. Training documents in Russian were provided to participants and could be used as TB guidelines pending printing of the Tajik TB guidelines. Nurses received a three-day training course. Two laboratory courses of 5 days were delivered for 10 doctors and 13 laboratory technicians from the same areas.

The International Federation of the Red Cross has started support to DOTS in 2002 by providing care to selected patients. These include vulnerable/disadvantaged persons such as single mothers. The program includes patient education as well as nutritional supplementation (a soup kitchen in Dushanbe) to provide food during the entire treatment program. Smear positive cases with limited income benefit from this support, which is an incentive for poor people to complete treatment. MERLIN conducts regular health education activities, including on TB, throughout the country.

Funding

According to the NTP 2000–2005, the estimated annual cost of the program is US$1.72 million. There is a huge unmet need for funding and a vast lack of local resources, including within prisons. Therefore, the Country Coordination Committee has submitted a grant proposal for TB to the GFATM, but this was not yet funded. The most pressing needs are the following:

- National TB surveillance system
- TB/MDR TB prevalence surveys
- DOTS program evaluation, including on treatment effectiveness
- Scaling up DOTS strategy implementation, including in prisons
- Training on DOTS (including publication of training and educational materials)
- Public awareness campaign
- Lab equipment
- Vehicles for DOT supervision
- TB drug management
- Food for TB patients

TABLE 24. PARTNER ACTIVITY ON TB PREVENTION AND CONTROL IN TAJIKISTAN

Partner	TB control program activity	Funding	Gap
WHO	Technical assistance Training including fellowship, conferences, meetings (together with HOPE) DOTS Program supervision (with HOPE, MINISTRY OF HEALTH) Laboratory and x-ray supplies for I year	$14,000 for 2002–2004	Microscopes Buffer stock lab supply
GDF	TB Drugs (incl. distribution costs) for DOTS pilot areas		Transport TB drugs for non DOTS areas
HOPE/ USAID	Set up an office in Dushanbe in 2001 Establishing a TB team through public education activities 3 year DOTS project in Dushanbe and Leninsky rayon to implement: DOTS program management together with WHO, MINISTRY OF HEALTH health staff training on DOTS Provision of equipment for the reference laboratory	$70,000	Transport (2 cars at central level, I car in Leninsky)
CDC/USAID	Conduct regular training workshops and on-site training for laboratory technicians from Dushanbe, Machenton and Leninsky		
IFRC/World Food Program	Activities designed to raise case detection and cure rates, including IEC/advocacy	$30,000 $ I/day/ patient for 100 cases.	Food for TB patients
Gov. India	TB Drugs for Machenton hospital for 600 patients coming from outside Dushanbe in 2001		
MERLIN	Assessment of TB laboratories in Dushanbe and Khatlon Oblast, and TB hospitals and programs in Dushanbe and Khatlon Oblast		

CHAPTER 7

COUNTRY PROFILE:
TURKMENISTAN

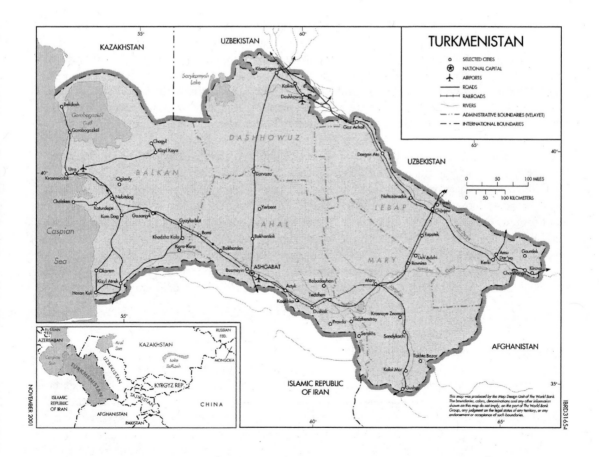

T urkmenistan has a population of approximately 5 million people, with about 46 percent in the age group16–45 years. The country is rich in oil and natural gas, and it has great potential for economic and social development. No reliable information is available on poverty. Physical infrastructure and social services are extremely underdeveloped, and the country suffers from a chronic water shortage.

HIV/AIDS Epidemiological Profile

Little data are available on HIV/AIDS in Turkmenistan. Officially, there have been only two reported cases of HIV/AIDS, both of whom are foreigners (one from Ukraine and the other from Africa), and one of whom would have died. The Turkmen State News Service reported in 2001 that, "AIDS is not a problem in Turkmenistan due to the success of the governmental anti-AIDS measures." However, data on IDU and STIs suggest a risk scenario similar to that of other ECA countries, with high rates of IDU and growing rates of STIs. Furthermore, with UNAIDS assistance, the Government has just carried out a situation assessment that may drastically change information on HIV/AIDS. However, the Government has not made the results public so far.

According to available official statistics, the number of drug users in Turkmenistan increased 400 percent in 1995 to 1997 alone. Turkmenistan currently has about 6,000 registered drug users, 95 percent of whom are male, but UNODCCP estimates that the real number is more than 50,000, of which 15 percent are IDUs. In addition, approximately 50 percent of the prisoners in Turkmenistan are thought to be IDUs. The risk of HIV transmission among these risk group members is evidently high, as limited surveillance data reported by UNAIDS show that as many as 80 percent of IDUs have Hepatitis B antigen, suggesting widespread needle and syringe sharing.

According to UNICEF (2002), the incidence of STIs nationwide was of 80/100,000 in 2000. Furthermore, syphilis incidence increased seven-fold over the period 1992 to 1998, and the Ministry of Health suggests that only 30 percent of syphilis and gonorrhea cases are reported through official surveillance systems. It is likely that most STI cases are treated outside the government health system for reasons of confidentiality, access, and annonymity, and it is not clear how many of these high-risk persons are screened for HIV, if at all. Given the risks of HIV transmission through evidently widespread risky sexual behavior, the lack of contact tracing and screening for STIs, and the added risk of HIV transmission through ulcerative STIs, the number of HIV cases is likely already higher than two in this country. Incidence would be expected to increase exponentially in the near future as in other Central Asian republics.

High average drug prices (one gram of heroin costs $70) may have contributed to relatively low demand and low IDU usage in the past. In addition, local researchers believe that the predominant form of drug use (heroin and opium) is through smoking instead of injection. Thus, there may be relatively lower risk for many drug-addicted persons in Turkmenistan, but the high rates of Hepatitis B antigen in some populations of drug users suggests that significant needle sharing does occur. Clearly, more research on behavior patterns among the highly vulnerable IDU population is needed in order to accurately characterize the status of the HIV/AIDS epidemic in Turkmenistan. To date, political and social influences appear to have inhibited the epidemiological investigations needed for this characterization.

Strategies, Policies, and Legal Framework

Government strategies have focused on drug supply interdiction in Turkmenistan, although the international press reports many local problems with this approach. Turkmenistan has an extensive border with Afghanistan (the source of most heroin and opium), but the Government claims a successful border strategy involving border troops and Ministry of Interior agents. Clearly, this interdiction strategy is not completely successful in deterring drug use; economic forces, both on the supply side as well as on the demand side, where poverty and destitution facilitate drug use, can overwhelm such a strategy.

Although the President signed a Law on Prevention of HIV/AIDS in 1991, this law has been revised and is under consideration by the Parliament. The Government has adopted a National Program for HIV/AIDS for 1999–2003. The main goals of the program are to prevent the spread of HIV/AIDS through blood product transfusion and unsafe sex. Program coordination is the responsibility of an Inter-Ministerial Task Force led by the Ministry of Health, National AIDS Center, and the STIs Dispensary. In addition to the line ministries, the committee includes representatives from the Democratic Party of Turkmenistan, Women's Union, Youth Union, National Centre of Trade Unions, and the National Society of Red Crescent. The plan is implemented by all involved parties with active assistance from the UNAIDS TG, but no monitoring and evaluation data on program results are available. The National HIV/AIDS Program includes five main areas:

- Definition of AIDS/STI policies, including revision of current legislation and a multi-sectoral approach;
- Early prevention of HIV/AIDS;
- Prevention of blood born transmission, including prevention of IDU;
- Prevention of sexual transmission, through safer sexual behavior, provision of condoms, and availability of STIs information, counseling, and treatment;
- Prevention of mother-to-child transmission through provision of information and increased use of condoms; and
- Support to people living with HIV/AIDS

The Ministry of Health has also developed a National Reproductive Health Strategy in which HIV prevention is addressed, and within this strategy, it plans to adopt the syndromic approach for STIs as recommended by the WHO. The AIDS National Program also seeks revision of drug use legislation. Drug users caught consuming drugs are only administratively fined by the police, but those who commit criminal offenses theoretically are referred for medical treatment of their drug addiction. Prostitution is illegal in Turkmenistan, and the first time a CSW is arrested, he/she is fined; if arrested a second time within the same year, he/she is imprisoned. The extent to which the CSW and IDU risk groups overlap is unknown. Given the social disruption and economic pressures on these risk groups, it is clear that more data are needed on their behaviors and potential to spread blood born infections such as HIV through the general population.

Surveillance Needs and Additional Studies

UNODCCP carried out a HIV/AIDS Rapid Assessment in Turkmenistan, but officially sanctioned data are not yet available from this study. UNICEF is also carrying out a baseline assessment of knowledge, attitudes, and behavior among youth. The National AIDS Program plans to develop sentinel surveillance among high risk groups such as IDUs and CSWs, and UNAIDS has supported the introduction of information technology for monitoring HIV/AIDS and STIs. However, few technological resources are available at the regional (Velayat) level. In addition to establishing sentinel surveillance, UNAIDS TG partners recommend evaluation studies on the impact of IEC measures implemented through Ministry of Health, hospitals, outpatient centers, and schools regarding HIV/AIDS and reproductive health. In Turkmenistan, there seems to be a significant lack of information about the extent of the HIV/AIDS epidemic and its antecedent risk conditions. Part of this appears to be a function of Government secrecy, but technical resources and lack of training appear to impede progress in this area.

Vulnerable and Highly Vulnerable Groups

The UNAIDS TG has provided active support to the implementation of the AIDS National Program, including training of government staff and NGOs and education of young people. Support has been provided to young vulnerable women who engage in casual and commercial sex work, through peer education, condom promotion, and access to appropriate health care. A competitive grant mechanism to support NGOs that carry out training and outreach activities has been established.

Various groups have provided syringes and bleach in Dashoguz, and syringes in three prisons (in Ahal Region), which is justified in the context of hepatitis prevention and not HIV/AIDS. UNFPA has been distributing more than one million condoms per year, and in 2002, it also supplied 5,000 women with condoms. The management of condom distribution has changed. Previously, they were distributed through the National Mother and Child Center, but now condoms are distributed through the National Reproductive Health Centers and the National AIDS Centers. UNFPA has also started working with the Army, having organized trainings with soldiers to discuss reproductive health issues, contraception, STIs, and urological diseases.

The Ministry of Health carries out HIV/AIDS education activities, but these have not been evaluated. The Youth Union has a TV Channel (Yaslik), which can be used for health promotion and education programs. In 1998, when the UNAIDS started activities in Turkmenistan, discussion of HIV/AIDS in the media was prohibited, but since then an extensive media awareness campaign has been implemented. UNAIDS and UNICEF have been assisting the development·of public awareness regarding HIV/AIDS and condom promotion, especially among youth. UNICEF works with youth and has a program known as Adolescent Lifestyle, which addresses issues of lifestyle, risk behavior, STI, HIV/AIDS, and substance abuse by advocating access to information; this program provides life skills training in schools and to out-of-school youth through various youth clubs.

Preventive, Diagnostic, and Treatment Issues

Given the officially reported data on HIV/AIDS, it is surprising to find that Turkmenistan has six AIDS centers (one national and five regional in each Velayat). Anonymous testing centers with hot lines have been established, and the country has 27 diagnostic laboratories that may perform HIV serologic testing. STIs services are provided at six STI hospitals and a few general hospital departments, and venereologists work in health polyclinics at the rural level. The Ministry of Health has established three STI Centers which provide condoms free of charge. The Center for Dermatology and Venereal Diseases opened a special center for reproductive health, which deals with all sexually transmitted infections, including HIV/AIDS. There is also a Reproductive Health Center for Men, since a large number of them have STIs and infertility, which also provides information on HIV/AIDS. The Ministry of Health is planning to adopt the syndromic approach for STIs, although it is considered very expensive. There are also 3,000 family group practices, which the Ministry of Health considers could become engaged on HIV/AIDS prevention activities. No information is available on anti-retroviral treatment or on MTCT prevention.

NGO and Partner Activities

In Turkmenistan, the local NGOs are called Community Based Organizations (CBOs). There are officially five CBOs, with other CBOs operating under the umbrella of those five. The only international NGOs working in Turkmenistan are Counterpart Consortium (funded by USAID) and MSF. The UNAIDS TG includes UNAIDS, UNFPA, UNICEF, UNDP, and USAID. The TG activities include:

- Ensuring political commitment through the adoption of a National Strategy (up to 2010);
- Supporting the National HIV/AIDS Program;
- Implementing an IEC Campaign for children, youth, and women;
- Promoting healthy lifestyles;
- Reducing the risk of vulnerable groups: IDUs, CSWs and MSM through outreach work.

Partner organizations report that constant changes in Government poses special challenges to the continuity of HIV/AIDS prevention work in Turkmenistan. It has been difficult to implement activities through the educational system, and work in prisons has faced constant changes in system leadership. Therefore, UNAIDS TG partners consider it essential to engage in a public communication campaign to increase Government political commitment and public awareness in general about HIV/AIDS.

Funding

No official information on public expenditures on HIV/AIDS and STI programs is available in Turkmenistan. However, the AIDS National Program estimates that the cost of implementing the work plan in 1999–2003 was $2.75 million, of which $1.7 million was for prevention of HIV transmission in blood products and unsafe sex (condom distribution), and $1 million for support to PLWHA. Last year, the Ministry of Health submitted to donors a $600,000 proposal on HIV/AIDS. The proposal would include establishing an electronic network for disease surveillance (including HIV sentinel surveillance), building the capacity of CBOs, and a public communications campaign.

USAID provided $51,000 for HIV/AIDS prevention work in Turkmenistan in 2000, and it has allocated $200,000 for these activities for 2002–2003. The Asian Development Bank has been assisting the activity of the UNAIDS TG on IEC and training family doctors and nurses on counseling regarding HIV/AIDS. UNICEF has been implementing a four-year, US$4.3 million program (2000–2004) that includes HIV/AIDS prevention activities among youth.

Tuberculosis Epidemiological Profile

According to the WHO Health for All Database, the incidence of TB in Turkmenistan has increased almost by 50 percent during the 1990s, from 64/100,000 population in 1990 to 97 in 1999; between 1991 and 1998, TB mortality also increased from 17/100,000 to 28. However, these data differ from those reported by Turkmen sources (Table 25). These official statistics show that the TB incidence rate recently decreased 6 percent, from 84/100,000 in 1999 to 79 in 2001. This figure is inconsistent with the increase in mortality and incidence noted by WHO during the 1990s, suggesting inefficient TB case finding and notification. Furthermore, although data on TB in prisons are not available, TB rates are thought to be extremely high in these institutions. Unconfirmed reports suggest that prisons house 30 percent of all TB patients in Turkmenistan, and due to chronic overcrowding, many of these are annually released through amnesties. This situation, then, would serve as an epidemiologic pump to raise the real burden of TB, although, again, little data are available on the follow-up of released prisoners with TB. Continuity between prison and civilian TB control systems is lacking.

TABLE 25. REPORTED TUBERCULOSIS INCIDENCE AND MORTALITY RATES IN TURKMENISTAN

	1997	1998	1999	2000	2001
Incidence Rate	72.3	78.8	84.1	82.3	78.7
Mortality Rate	10.3	12.4	13.6	14.2	14.0

Source: Turkmenistan State Medical School, Department of Tuberculosis

On a regional data level, the burden of TB is better represented (Table 26). Incidence has increased from 2000 to 2001 in two of the oblasts, but mortality rates have remained relatively unchanged during these two years. The total number of TB cases reported in Turkmenistan is slightly higher for 2001 than 2000 (14,285 versus 14,171).

Strategies, Policies, and Legal Framework

Overall, there is still insufficient Government commitment to TB control in Turkmenistan. The Government recognizes that the TB problem is important, and it welcomes foreign financial and technical assistance. However, there is little open discussion about the true magnitude of the problem, and national funding for TB control is inadequate. The Ministry of Health plans to achieve 100 percent coverage of new cases with DOTS strategy by the end of 2003, including in prisons. Although DOTS pilot projects are underway, a National TB control program is still being prepared.

TABLE 26. TB IN TURKMEN REGIONS

Region	New Cases 2000	New Cases 2001	Incidence rate 2000	Incidence rate 2001	Prevalent Cases 2000	Prevalent Cases 2001	Prevalence rate 2000	Prevalence rate 2001	Number of Deaths 2000	Number of Deaths 2001	Mortality rate 2000	Mortality rate 2001
Dashoguz	1174	1087	112.6	103	3876	3583	372	339	141	133	13.5	12.6
Ashkhabad	530	662	91.8	114.2	1817	1944	315	335	130	140	22.5	24.1
Balkan	353	376	89.9	95.0	1182	1163	301	294	75	72	19.1	18.2
Leban	740	601	73.7	59.1	2753	2862	274	282	133	114	13.2	11.2
Mary	692	751	62.0	66.4	2884	3048	258	270	135	150	12.1	13.3
Akhal	478	356	69.9	51.4	1659	1685	243	243	71	72	10.4	10.4
Total	3967	3833	82.3	78.7	14171	14285	294	293	685	681	14.2	14.0

Source: Turkmenistan State Medical School, Department of Tuberculosis.

Access to services is difficult for most patients, and a recent decision to move the National TB Clinic several miles away from the capital (Ashgabad) will likely further decrease access to TB services for urban residents.

TABLE 27. TB TREATMENT SUCCESS RATES, DASHOGUZ DOTS PILOT PROJECT

Patient category	N	Treatment success rate*	Death rate**	Failure rate***	Default rate****
New smear positive pulmonary	124	73%	4.8%	8.9%	12.9%
New smear negative pulmonary	134	87%	6.7%	0	4.5%
Re-treatment smear positive pulmonary	398	68%	6.8%	9.8%	12.6%
Re-treatment smear negative pulmonary	276	93%	1.1%	0.7%	4.3%
Extra-pulmonary	290	92%	1.7%	0	5.5%

Source: MSF (2002). Summary of tuberculosis treatment and outcomes for the Aral Sea Area TB Program.
* The success rate is the percentage of all patients who have the outcome of cured and have completed treatment.
** The death rate is the percentage of patients who die from any cause during treatment.
*** The failure rate is the percentage of patients who remain or become sputum smear positive at 5 months or more of treatment. A high failure rate suggests a poor DOTS program with low adherence to treatment or a high rate of drug-resistant TB that is difficult to cure with first line TB drugs.
**** A patient is classified as a defaulter if treatment is interrupted for at least two consecutive months.

Surveillance Needs and Additional Studies

There is no regular monitoring of DOTS pilot project implementation. Prison TB cases are not reported, and therefore these cases are not even included in official statistics. However, an NGO (MSF) conducts regular evaluation of treatment outcomes in the Dashoguz DOTS pilot region (Table 27). Drug-susceptibility testing is not yet regularly available, but to quantify the problem of MDRTB and adapt treatment regimens, MSF initiated a rigorous study of drug susceptibility for new TB cases in July 2001. Preliminary results from the study suggest rates of drug resistance, including multi-drug resistance that are among the highest in the world (MSF, unpublished data presented at the International Union against Tuberculosis and Lung Disease (IUATLD) annual conference in Montreal, 2002).

Preventive, Diagnostic, and Treatment Issues

The Ministry of Health recognizes TB as an important public health problem, and it approved the implementation of DOTS pilots in several oblasts. Population coverage with DOTS was aimed at

70 percent, but current coverage is only 34 percent. The DOTS strategy has not yet been implemented in prisons, which are under the administration of the Ministry of Internal Affairs, and this
complicates a truly national approach to TB control. The DOTS strategy implementation started in
2000 in two sites of Dashoguz region, with assistance from MSF, and in Ashgabat and Turkmenbashi with WHO technical assistance, CDC training, and financial and technical support from
Project HOPE/USAID. By April 2002, MSF had covered all Dashoguz rayons with DOTS.

However, DOTS pilot programs have not been very successful: a treatment success rate of
73 percent was reported for new smear sputum positive TB patients registered in Dashoguz in
2000. This is due to very high default (13 percent) and failure (9 percent) rates. A high drug resistance level may be the cause for the high failure rate. No official data are available on treatment
success rates for non-DOTS areas.

In DOTS pilot areas, case finding is passive and diagnosis is based on smear microscopy with
some use of radiography. Inpatient care is provided in TB facilities during the first two months of
intensive treatment, followed by outpatient treatment provided by general health staff for four
months. There is monitoring during treatment, and follow-up occurs through local health facilities. Standardized multi-drug therapy is employed. In Dashoguz, therapy is directly observed in
the inpatient phase only, as ambulatory patients return to their rural homes that are far from
health posts. TB workers manage directly observed therapy in the community-based continuation
phase as well.

Public awareness about TB is low; for example, there is a widespread belief that TB is a heredi-
tary disease, and therefore TB patients are highly stigmatized. There is a lack of funding, equipment, and supplies to fully implement a National program. The Ministry of Health supported the
pilot program by renovating the laboratory at the Central TB Hospital, which opened in June
2000. Partner organizations consider that there is no real commitment to provide laboratory
equipment and training, updating treatment protocols, and providing TB drugs outside the central
level. Quality smear bacteriology services are only limited to pilot DOTS areas. Although a request
for TB drugs was approved by the Global Drug Fund, no drugs have been received yet. Recent
decisions about the movement of the Central TB Research Hospital outside the capital may complicate coordination of treatment and laboratory services. The DOTS approach is now included in
the National Medical Board Certification Examinations.

National TB drug production has been established, including combination TB drugs. The
Government procures all TB drugs from the locally based "Ajantafarma" pharmaceutical company
(supported 80 percent by public funding), but funding for procurement of TB drugs is still insufficient. Production is not GMP certified, and quality is questionable as dosages are inconsistent with
WHO recommendations.

NGO and Partner Activities

NGO involvement in TB control in Turkmenistan is only modest outside of DOTS pilot areas.
The International Committee of the Red Cross is planning to work with TB patients who default
on treatment, with medical students involved as treatment supervisors on a voluntary basis.

As for multi-national health organizations, there appear to be problems in cooperation or
communication with the Government. The WHO Regional Advisor, based in Almaty, provides
technical assistance, but WHO has not been able to obtain data on TB from the Ministry of
Health. The reasons for this lack of coordination are not clear.

Project HOPE/USAID activities in Turkmenistan began in 2000. The program based on the
DOTS strategy delivered lab equipment for Ashgabat and Turkmenbashi, the two selected pilot
sites, including binocular microscopes, incubators, centrifuges, refrigerators, medical ware, and lab
reagents. Project HOPE also provided anti-TB drugs for 1,000 patients. To date, Project HOPE
staff working with the Turkmenistan Medical University TB faculty has provided training for 470
TB specialists, primary health care physicians, and other health professionals in Ashgabat. In 2001,
the second pilot site opened in Turkmenbashi, and training was provided to all medical staff. CDC

provides monitoring of the Central TB laboratory and regional TB laboratories to ensure that quality assurance procedures are in place.

MSF has been involved in TB control in Turkmenistan for three years. The MSF program in the Dashoguz region consists of training health care workers, and the provision of drugs and lab equipment. Efforts were also made to improve managerial skills among Ministry of Health staff; include children in the DOTS implementation; sustain laboratory quality control; and to improve tracing of treatment defaulters. Although Project HOPE and MSF trained many health care workers on DOTS, many more trained staff will be needed to expand DOTS to the entire country.

Funding

No information is available on public funding for TB control. Additional efforts and funding are necessary to increase Government commitment to TB control and public awareness about TB; upgrade surveillance and carry out drug resistance surveys; and to improve the quality and supply of TB drugs, lab supplies, and office equipment.

CHAPTER 8

COUNTRY PROFILE: UZBEKISTAN

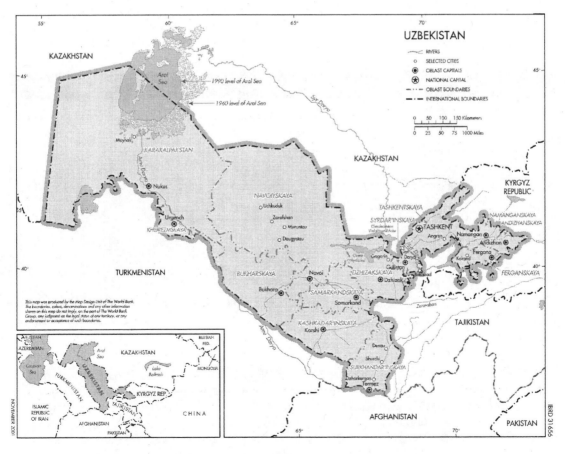

Uzbekistan is the most populous country in Central Asia, with 25 million persons. More than 25 percent of the population is between 15–29 years of age. The country has a GDP per capita of almost $3,000, but over 60 percent of the population lives below the official level of poverty ($4/day). Uzbekistan is an Islamic country, which has been ruled since the breakup of the Soviet Union by a President and a centralized Government.

HIV/AIDS Epidemiological Profile

The HIV epidemic in Uzbekistan is still in a nascent stage, but Uzbekistan has all the conditions for rapid spread of HIV infection. While only 51 cases had been identified in the first ten years of the epidemic (1989–1998), almost 800 cases were registered by the end of 2001, and 2,209 cases by end of April 2003; of these cases 84 died. However, according to official definitions, HIV positive patients with TB are not diagnosed as having AIDS, thus contributing to an underreporting of HIV/AIDS (TB is the most common opportunistic infection among HIV-infected persons.) About 55 percent of cases of HIV/AIDS are reported among people under age 30 years.

According to the Ministry of Health, injection drug use accounts for the majority (63 percent) of HIV infections, as in other countries in the region, but the proportion of cases of heterosexual transmission is growing. Of concern is the high number of cases of unknown origin (about 25 percent). About 84 percent of HIV cases are among men, and two-thirds are among young people aged 15–34. More than 50 percent of cases are among prisoners. The highest number of cases has been identified in Tashkent. In April 2002, there were about 350–360 infected people in Tashkent City, another 350–360 in Tashkent Oblast, and about 40 each in Ferghana and Surkhan-Darya regions. An outbreak of HIV was registered in Yangiyul (near Tashkent) with over 200 HIV cases, of which 90 percent were IDUs. It is an industrial zone and, due to economic reforms, many plants have closed, leaving many young people unemployed.

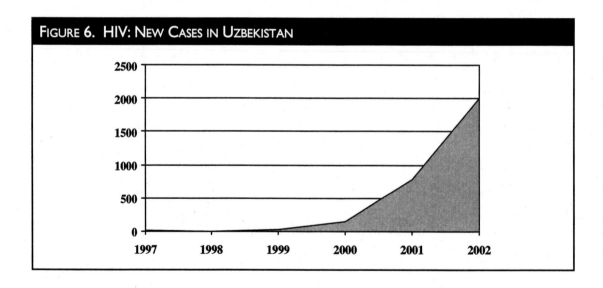

FIGURE 6. HIV: NEW CASES IN UZBEKISTAN

The number of registered drug users is around 25,000, but the UN estimates that the country has at least 60,000 drug users, 60–70 percent of whom would be injecting drug users. In the 1980s, there were 2,000 registered drug users; in 1995, there were 6,000 registered drug users, but today there are 18,000 registered outside prisons and 7,000 identified in prisons. According to surveys conducted by UNAIDS, there are about 12,000 IDUs in Tashkent City alone; 1,800–2,000 in Yangiyul City; 10,000–10,5000 in Samarkand City; and 1,300 in Jizzak City.

These areas are on the crossroads of drug traffic routes from Tajikistan and Afghanistan, where opium and heroin are produced. Since September 11, 2001, the frontiers with Afghanistan have been opened. The drugs coming from Afghanistan go through Uzbekistan to Russia by railroad. While older generations commonly smoked hashish, younger generations have shifted to injecting heroin. One region that does not have any HIV cases is Karakalpakstan, which is attributed to the fact that drug users from this region still mainly smoke drugs instead of injecting them. As a result, HIV/AIDS is regarded as a problem of injecting drug users, which significantly stigmatizes this vulnerable group.

The proportion of IDU-related cases appears to be declining, however, while the rate of infection through heterosexual contact appears to be rapidly increasing, representing currently over 12 percent of infected cases. Migration to Tashkent has increased, accompanied by increasing prostitution; many of these women also become drug users. An assessment of men who have sex with men carried out in 1998 mentions that homosexual behavior is a common practice in Uzbekistan (Oostvogels and Mikkelsen 1998). Alarmingly, there have also been unconfirmed reports that some poorly equipped hospitals are part of the HIV transmission process through nosocomial transmission. This is compounded by claims that the blood supply in places is not adequately screened for organisms found in HIV, Hepatitis B, and Hepatitis C.

According to official statistics, 1.2 percent of IDUs (over 18,000 tested), 0.01 percent of CSW (over 15,000 tested), and 0.4 percent of prisoners (over 65,000 tested) were HIV positive in 2001. However, sentinel surveillance in Tashkent indicates a 46 percent prevalence rate among IDUs in Tashkent City.[10] Isolated cases of HIV infection have also been reported in MSM, blood donors, patients with STIs, pregnant women, and newborns (3 cases in 2000–2001). According to the AIDS Center, of 360 people tested in 3 Trust Points, 45 percent were HIV positive, while results from a second study showed that only 20 percent

TABLE 28. HIV/AIDS IN UZBEKISTAN			
	1995	2000	2002
AIDS deaths			84
AIDS cases			25
HIV estimated cases			6,000
HIV registered cases	51		2,209*
HIV among IDUs (registered cases)			
Syphilis cases		73.5	
Registered drug users			25,000
Estimated # IDUS			100,000
Estimated # CSW			20,000
Estimated # MSM			15,000

Source: Ministry of Health. HIV cases refers to end of April 2003.

were infected. A rapid assessment of IDUs carried out in Tashkent in 1998 showed that over 90 percent were male and that the majority were young people aged 18–30 years (Busel etal. 1998). Almost 70 percent of IDUs were unemployed. Another rapid assessment carried out in Samarkand in 2001 showed that, among those who tested positive for HIV, almost 90 percent were male, 60 percent were young people under the age of 30, and the majority were unemployed (Zaripova etal. 2001).

Unsafe sexual behavior has increased, attested to by a high prevalence of STIs, compounding the risks for HIV spread. In 2001, Uzbekistan had 221 syphilis cases per 100,000 pregnant women, not usually considered a vulnerable group. However, this is 10 times the reported prevalence in the general population. One out of six CSWs who visited STIs services had syphilis. Rapid assessments of CSWs were carried out in Tashkent in 1997 (Thomas) and 2001 (Oostvogels). In 1997, the assessments estimated that there were 5,000 sex workers and 250,000 clients in the capital city. CSWs try to hide from authorities as indicated by the fact that only 180 sex workers were

---

10. CCM (2003). GFATM grant proposal. Tashkent: Republican Emergency Anti-epidemic Commission for HIV/AIDS and TB.

registered in Tashkent. This is despite the fact that 3,870 CSWs were tested for STIs in 1996, and over 15,000 were tested for HIV/AIDS by the AIDS Center in 2002.

Condoms are readily available from kiosks and are affordable for some CSWs at about 50 cents each. However, the majority of the CSWs, with ages varying from 13–30 years, do not use condoms, and 30 percent are IDUs. The majority of clients refuse to use condoms, particularly Uzbeks who are reportedly even more reluctant than foreigners to use condoms. However, other CSWs would be spending about 10 percent of what they earn from a client on a condom. The Uzbek Health Examination Survey indicates that only 2 percent of married women reported using condoms, but this percentage increased to 27 percent among unmarried women; only 1 percent of married men reported using condoms, while 39 percent of unmarried men reported condom use (Ministry of Health 2003).

A survey of 3,600 young people (15–24 years) throughout Uzbekistan has indicated that 44 percent of young males have sexual activity but only 23 percent use any form of contraception (Uzbek Association on Reproductive Health/IPPR 2001). This survey also indicates that they are learning little or nothing about how HIV infection is transmitted and prevented through school educational programs designed to provide this information. According to the survey, 50 percent of young people consider that there is no risk of being infected by HIV and another 40 percent are not even aware of this risk. UNICEF (2002) reports that 43 percent of young people aged 14–17 are aware of condom use as a means of HIV prevention. However, among women aged 30–49, the proportion decreases to 35 percent, and among young women aged 15–29, the proportion further decreases to 26 percent. The (UHES) reports that 90 percent of female respondents and 95 percent of male respondents have heard of AIDS, but only about 60 percent of women and 80 percent of men believe that there is a way to avoid AIDS.

Strategies, Policies, and Legal Framework

Commitment to prevent further spread of HIV/AIDS is shown by the following: the approval of an AIDS Law and of the HIV/AIDS National Program; the Government approval of an appropriate Strategy[11] prepared with assistance from UNAIDS; a functioning UN-Theme Group; the establishment of more than 200 Trust Points throughout the country; and requests for grants from the GFATM and IDA to contribute to assist in addressing the burgeoning epidemic.

The Government is also committed to the fight against IDU, and it has signed all international conventions against drug trafficking. A Special State Committee headed by the Prime Minister has been set up to tackle the struggle against drug trafficking, with special units in the Ministry of Health and Ministry of Internal Affairs. The Inter-ministerial Committee on Drug Abuse includes the Ministries of Interior, Defense, Education, Health, Social Protection, and Labor. In July 2002, the Government of Uzbekistan hosted the regional Conference on Drug Trafficking and Use.

Strategic planning on HIV/AIDS was initiated by the UN-AIDS Theme Group, which is currently chaired by the World Bank, and it has been supported by the Government. In addition, the Ministry of Health has been cooperating with UN agencies and donors on implementation of HIV/AIDS activities. The Ministry of Internal Affairs has also been cooperating with the Soros Foundation/OSI on the implementation of HIV/AIDS activities in prisons. The recently approved HIV/AIDS Strategy aims to:

■ Encourage a multi-sectoral approach in the implementation of the HIV/AIDS Strategy with the involvement of relevant line ministries such as Ministries of Health, Internal Affairs, Education, and Finance, and UN agencies and NGOs.?

---

11. Interdepartamental Working Group on HIV/AIDS (2002). Strategic Program on Counteraction to HIV/AIDS epidemic expansion in the Republic of Uzbekistan. Tashkent: Government of Uzbekistan.

- Strengthen targeted interventions for high-risk populations, which are critical to reversing the HIV/AIDS epidemic in Uzbekistan.
- Strengthen the management structure and implementation capacity to ensure the sustainability of the National Program on HIV/AIDS and STIs.

The Strategy considers the following as factors conducive to the spread of HIV infection in Uzbekistan: 1) insufficient governance to fight the epidemic; 2) weak multi-sectoral coordination; 3) high susceptibility of groups of the population in which the infection is concentrated; 4) incomplete observance of human rights and freedoms related to HIV/AIDS; and 5) insufficient focus on prevention activities, care and treatment, and support to PLWHA. In reality, there is poor interministerial coordination, and the Government was reluctant to approve the HIV/AIDS Strategy and proposals for funding to the GFATM out of religious and cultural concerns.

Illegal purchase and storage of drugs is prosecuted as a criminal offense, and drug replacement therapy is not yet legal in Uzbekistan. CSWs are prosecuted by law, and MSM are also subject to criminal prosecution. The Law on AIDS further contributes to stigmatization of HIV infected people, which provides an additional incentive for highly vulnerable groups to avoid testing.

Surveillance Needs and Additional Studies

Uzbekistan has 14 AIDS centers and 90 laboratories for HIV diagnosis. The AIDS Center publishes quarterly reports on HIV/AIDS. UNAIDS has carried several rapid situation assessments in Tashkent since 1998. ODCCP is carrying out a survey on drug abuse in Uzbekistan. CDC is carrying out a HIV prevalence survey in Tashkent, and the results should be available in 2003. USAID in cooperation with CDC is providing equipment for the AIDS laboratories and training in sentinel surveillance.

The National AIDS Center laboratory has identified thousands of HIV positive cases by ELISA, which need to be confirmed by Western Blot. Rapid assessments were carried out on IDUs in five regions (Tashkent City, Sukhandaria, Samarkhand, Gizak, Tashkent), and the blood in syringes from three Trust Points was tested.

Vulnerable and Highly Vulnerable Groups

Since the Uzbek Parliament passed a law on prevention of HIV/AIDS in 2000, Trust Points have been opened throughout Uzbekistan. These points are expected to provide counseling, testing, and free syringes, condoms, and information brochures. After the successful establishment of pilot Trust Points, the Minister of Health decreed that each oblast AIDS Center should set up at least one Trust Point providing anonymous and confidential testing and counseling for IDUs. Recognizing this initiative as best practice, UNAIDS reports that this is the first initiative by national authorities to implement trust points nationwide in Central Asia. The Ministry of Health has reported that the number of registered HIV cases actually decreased by 38 percent in areas where Trust Points are active.

The Government supports the harm reduction approach, and it has decided to increase the number of Trust points from 50 to 230. Currently, about 200 Trust Points are functioning throughout the country, up from 3 that were opened in 2000. In Tashkent City, there are 10 Trust Points, which distribute 800 to 1,000 needles daily, the same number that is distributed in all other oblasts. Volunteers work with the drug users who come to the trust points and speak with them confidentially. Fees for volunteers, syringes, and other supplies are paid by Government or are provided by the Soros Foundation/OSI. However, the Trust Points are frequently out of condoms, and health care workers work in cooperation with law enforcement bodies, which exercise repressive practices over groups at risk.

There is a prison pilot project on HIV/AIDS prevention in the Chirchik prison. Prisons usually isolate HIV positive prisoners, which has led to revolts in some prisons due to isolation. The Government has arranged a study tour to Karaganda, to observe HIV/AIDS prevention work in prisons in Kazakhstan. HIV/AIDS prevention work is also taking place in the army and information materials geared towards soldiers have been prepared.

The Government's current HIV prevention campaign, aimed almost exclusively at the IDU community, is considered a major barrier to preventing a broader epidemic. This approach is leading young people to think that the HIV/AIDS phenomenon does not affect them, but rather only marginalized people such as IDUs. Although an educational program has been developed for schools, it has not yet been integrated in the compulsory curricula. IEC for out-of-school young people and a public awareness campaign through the mass media have not yet been developed.

UN agencies and USAID/CAR have been training mass media and raising public awareness on drug related issues. UNICEF has also been conducting an IEC strategy to raise awareness regarding drug abuse, safe sexual behavior, and HIV/AIDS and STIs for 40,000 people aged 13–20 years. PSI, with funding from USAID, has been implementing a condom social marketing campaign, in which condoms are distributed at a low price.

Preventive, Diagnostic, and Treatment Issues

The UN Office for Drug Control and Crime Prevention (UNODCCP) and the Government of Switzerland have assisted in the establishment of a network of narcological health centers for treatment of drug abuse. Soros Foundation/OSI and the International Harm Reduction Network (IHRD) support a policy for replacement therapy for treatment of drug abuse. Methadone is on the list of drugs not allowed into the country, but there are attempts to develop a pilot project on replacement therapy with methadone. Recently seven specialists spent a month in the United States studying the implementation of substitution therapy.

No information is available on treatment of opportunistic infections, and as a rule, HIV-infected people do not have access to antiretroviral treatment.

NGO and Partner Activities

There are numerous NGOs working on HIV/AIDS in Uzbekistan: Kamalot works with youth; Sabokh and Tiklal Avlot work with CSWs (2 projects); Anti-AIDS works with MSMs; and Mahala works with IDUs (2 projects). NGOs are mainly funded by international and bilateral agencies.

The UN Theme Group includes the Ministries of Health, Defense, and Interior, and World Bank, USAID, Soros Foundation/OSI, UNAIDS, UNDP, UNFP, UNICEF, UNDCP, WHO and NGOs. The TG has an integrated working plan, which includes a list of 29 NGOs involved in HIV/AIDS work in the country. USAID has been providing technical and financial support to HIV/AIDS prevention in Uzbekistan, including upgrades in surveillance and in the lab system, prevention of mother to child transmission and blood safety. The Soros Foundation/OSI has been supporting the establishment of Trust Points in cooperation with the AIDS Center. The International Harm Reduction Program (IHRP) is also involved in harm reduction and prevention of HIV/AIDS with financial support of USAID.

Funding

In 2001, 3.4 percent of total public expenditure was on health, which gives a spending per capita of less than $10. The Government has indicated a budget for the HIV/AIDS Program of $704,000 in 2003, and in addition $610,000 from donors. For the period of 2001–2003, UN agencies, USAID, and Soros Foundation/OSI have been providing over $1.5 million, and KfW has been providing DM5 million for family planning, including contraceptives and condoms. Although the Government supports the establishment of the Trust Points throughout the country, funding is insufficient to cover the needs, which have been estimated at about $40 million for four years. Therefore, the Government has applied to IDA, GFATM, and bilateral agencies for financial and technical support.

Recently, the Government started preparation for an AIDS component of a World Bank-financed project, which would be included in Health Project II. The AIDS Component would be financed by an IDA grant of about $2 million. The Ministry of Health and project team have agreed that the component would support the approval and implementation of the HIV/AIDS Strategy that the Ministry of Health prepared with assistance from UNAIDS and has been recently approved. The component would also complement activities that have been launched with support from the Government and donors.

The Ministry of Health has also submitted, with assistance from the UN-Theme Group, a grant proposal to the GFATM in the amount of $24 million, of which was granted $5 million. An Interministerial Committee, with participation of UN agencies and NGOs, would steer the implementation of the HIV/AIDS Strategy and the use of the funds available from the Government, IDA, GFATM, UN agencies, USAID, Soros Foundation/OSI, and other NGOs. The grant from the GFATM would cover other unfounded activities such as scaling up target prevention interventions throughout the country, treatment of opportunistic infections and AIDS, and palliative care.

Tuberculosis Epidemiological Profile

Even with reported rates of TB significantly lower than in Kazakhstan and the Kyrgyz Republic, Uzbekistan has the largest number of TB cases in the region. A very low percentage of notified pulmonary smear positive cases (expected value should be over 50 percent) suggests that the true dimensions of the TB problem may be about twice as high as reported. The TB situation has been worsening in Uzbekistan (Table 29); notification of new TB cases increased by almost two thirds (65 percent) in the last 10 years, and the death rate increased by one third (30 percent) in the last five years. The highest TB notification rate in 2000 was in Karakalpakstan (128/100,000), which is twice as high as the national rate of 65. In 2001, the TB reported incidence rate was 72.4/100,000 for a total of 18,106 new TB cases, and the death rate was 12.5.

TABLE 29. TUBERCULOSIS DETECTION, CASES, INCIDENCE, AND MORTALITY IN UZBEKISTAN										
	1992	1993	1994	1995	1996	1997	1998	1999	2000	2001
Cases notified	9,370	9,774	14,890	9,866	11,919	13,352	14,558	15,080	15,750	18,106
Notification rate	44	45	67	43	51	56	60	62	63	72.4
New cases ss+ pulmonary	NA	NA	7,487	2,735	3,350	3,388	3,504	3,977	3,825	4,664
Notification rate Ss+ cases pulmonary	NA	NA	34	12	14	14	15	16	15	NA
% pulmonary ss+ cases	NA	NA	50	28	28	25	24	26	24	NA
Notified death rate						9.6	11.1	10.7	11.5	12.5
Standardized death rate	12.57	14.59	14.57	16.25	17.94	18.08	19.45	NA	NA	NA

Source: WHO Global TB Control 2002; WHO HFA database 2002; CDC Central Asia Infectious Disease Network 2002

The TB problem in prisons is grave. The incidence of TB in prisons is estimated at over 3,000/100,000 population (2,000 patients have been annually diagnosed in a population of 64,000 prisoners). Up to half of all TB cases in the country may be in prisons. There are now about 30,000 prisoners with active TB in prisons, one out of each 10–12 inmates. Approximately 6,000 prisoners with active TB were released by an amnesty in 2001. Those who had completed TB treatment were released under the supervision of primary health care (PHC) services at the place of residence, and those who had not completed treatment were placed into hospitals until completing treatment.

Strategy, Policies, and Legal Framework

Government commitment to TB control is sufficient, but the Ministry of Health has limited resources to tackle the problem. The Government recognizes that a significant TB problem exists in the country, and has started working on the development of a strategic plan and revised national program for TB control. The Ministry of Health of Uzbekistan is supportive of the WHO TB control strategy DOTS. A coordination council for DOTS implementation in Uzbekistan has also been established. This Council is chaired by the first Deputy Minister of Health and includes representatives of relevant departments of the Ministry of Health, National TB Research Institute, regional TB facilities, and international and donor organizations. A national DOTS Center affiliated with the National TB Research Institute was established with assistance from Project HOPE. Pilot DOTS projects have started with support from WHO, KfW, USAID, Project HOPE, and MSF. The National Program aims to cover most of the country (except the Jizzak and Nawoi regions) by the end of the first quarter of 2003 with the DOTS approach. The Ministry of Health is searching for potential donors, and it has prepared a grant proposal to submit to the GFATM to extend the program to the two uncovered regions.

Surveillance Needs and Additional Studies

Currently, quarterly analysis of treatment results based on WHO definitions is limited to the DOTS pilot areas. The National TB Program envisages the establishment of a standardized reporting and recording system (assisted by CDC), allowing assessment of treatment results according to WHO guidelines. CDC has also been assisting the establishment of a quality assurance program for TB laboratories and laboratory training. CDC plans to develop and start implementation of the TB electronic surveillance case-based management program. Preliminary results from a drug susceptibility testing study conducted by MSF in Karakalpakstan and Khorezm suggest that rates of drug resistance, including multi-drug resistance, are among the highest in the world (Table 30).

TABLE 30. MULTIPLE DRUG RESISTANT TB (%) IN UZBEKISTAN		
	Primary MDR New cases (%)	Secondary MDR Re-treatment cases (%)
Karakalpakstan	11	40

Source: MSF unpublished data, 2002

Preventive, Diagnostic, and Treatment Issues

The Ministry of Health intends to cover most of the country with DOTS by the end of 2003, but it needs to identify additional funding. The DOTS Strategy has been implemented in Uzbekistan since 1998, with support from WHO, MSF, USAID, Project Hope, CDC and KfW. However, the program has expanded slowly, and therefore it is unlikely to have a tangible impact on TB control. In 2000, only 7 percent of the population was covered with DOTS, and treatment success for patients registered in 1998 and 1999 was below the WHO target of 85 percent (Tables 31 and 32). A very high failure rate should be a cause for concern and the role of drug resistance and HIV infection needs to be investigated. MSF has provided support to the development of pilot projects in Karakalpakstan, and DOTS expansion accelerated with assistance from Project HOPE in 10 additional pilot districts. KfW has provided grant funding for TB drugs and lab equipment.

The National TB Program emphasizes abandoning MMR screening for TB and extensive utilization of inpatient treatments. The program gives priority to passive case finding (detection of TB among symptomatic patients self reporting to health services, using sputum smear microscopy) and limits active case finding to examination of household members of a sputum smear positive TB patient. The program specifies establishment of reference laboratories to ensure quality assurance for TB detection and diagnosis. Inpatient treatment at existing TB facilities is mandatory for all new TB cases during at least 2–3 months of the intensive treatment phase. Inpatient treatment can be extended for patients who fail treatment and/or with low socio-economic status. The program plans involvement of primary health care at rayon level for provision of out-patient treatment for TB at the continuation phase.

TABLE 31. SUCCESS RATES FOR TB TREATMENT, KARAKALPAKSTAN DOTS PILOT AREA

Patient category	N	Treatment success rate*	Death rate**	Failure rate***	Default rate****
New smear positive pulmonary	287	76	3.8	11.1	9.1
New smear negative pulmonary	397	93	1.5	2.3	2.3
Re-treatment smear positive pulmonary	330	60	13.9	15.2	10.6
Re-treatment smear negative pulmonary	388	86	3.6	2.8	7.5
Extra-pulmonary	107	92	0.9	0	7.5

Source: MSF (2002). Summary of tuberculosis treatment and outcomes for the Aral Sea Area TB program. Medecins Sans Frontieres – Holland, ASA Program.
* The success rate is the percentage of all patients who have the outcome of cured and have completed treatment.
** The death rate is the percentage of patients who die from any cause during treatment.
*** The failure rate is the percentage of patients who remain or become sputum smear positive at 5 months or more of treatment. A high failure rate can indicate a poor DOTS program with low adherence to treatment or a high rate of drug-resistant TB that is difficult to cure with first line TB drugs.
**** A patient is classified as a defaulter if their treatment was interrupted for at least two consecutive months.

Treatment of TB is based on WHO recommended standardized short course chemotherapy regimens. In DOTS pilot areas, TB treatment (including TB drugs) is free for patients. In non-DOTS areas, treatment is officially free, but in fact patients often have to buy the drugs.

There is capacity at the National TB Research Institute to expand DOTS, including the National DOTS Center staffed by trainers trained by Project HOPE, and the network of TB facilities (dispensaries, sanatoria, laboratories) throughout the country. Uzbekistan has 256 TB facilities, with over 15,000 beds, and 1,500 TB specialists. However, more health staff needs to be trained on DOTS to scale-up its implementation. There is a vast lack of funds to procure TB drugs, lab equipment and supplies, and to publish training and patient educational materials.

Prisons in Uzbekistan are under the management of the Ministry of Internal Affairs. No DOTS program has yet been implemented in Uzbek prisons due to a lack of funding. However, representatives of prison management expressed willingness to implement DOTS-based TB control. Prison authorities have developed a concept document on TB control in prisons, and they submitted an application to Soros Foundation/OSI for a DOTS pilot project in one of the colonies.

TABLE 32. TREATMENT OUTCOMES FOR NEW SMEAR-POSITIVE CASES TREATED UNDER DOTS IN UZBEKISTAN

Year	Registered for treatment No. patients	Cured %	Completed %	Died %	Failed %	Default %	Transfer %	Success* %
1998	135	73	6	7	7	7	1	79
1999	74	65	14	7	14	1		78

*Cured + Completed.
Source: WHO (1999–2002). Global TB Control.

NGO and Partner Activities

WHO, KfW, MSF and USAID through Project HOPE and CDC, have been active on TB control in Uzbekistan (Table 33). KfW has provided lab equipment and Project HOPE has been delivering 100 binocular microscopes, other lab equipment and reagents, and computers to 10 pilot districts and to the National Reference Laboratory at the TB Institute since 2002. KfW has pledged DM 1,115 million for procurement of first line TB drugs for prisons until 2005, but no funding has been received so far. With funding from USAID, Project HOPE trained a total of 45 clinical and laboratory trainers and 1,250 health providers, including 500 TB physicians, more than 500 primary care physicians, 45 nurses, and 100 laboratory specialists. Project HOPE held and sponsored conferences/workshops in Uzbekistan, and organized study tours and trips to international conferences for health care leaders of the country. Clinical and laboratory experts provided medical consultations, regular monitoring, and technical assistance in developing policy documents, including the National TB DOTS Program. In 2000–2001, Laboratory training and laboratory equipment were provided with technical assistance from CDC. In addition, TB drugs were provided for treatment of

TABLE 33.   NGO AND PARTNER ACTIVITY ON TB IN UZBEKISTAN

Implementing agency	Funding Agency	Sites	Population Covered 2002	Area of activity
CDC	USAID	Nationwide	NA	Quality assurance of TB laboratories in pilots; Laboratory training; Implementation of TB electronic surveillance case-based management program
HOPE	USAID KFW	Ferghana Andijon Namangan Samarkand Urgut Syrdarya Yangiyer Tashkent	NA	DOTS training of health staff; Provision of TB drugs and lab equipment (1250 patients treated); Lab quality control; DOTS program monitoring
MSF	SIDA Holland KFW	Khorazm	2,211,675	DOTS training of health staff (2000 health staff trained); Provision of TB drugs and lab equipment (9641 patient treated and 22 laboratories upgraded); Managerial training for Ministry of Health staff; Lab quality control; DOTS program monitoring
KFW		Karakalpakstan Karakalpakstan Khorezm Tashkent Surkhondaryo Qashqadaryo Bukhara W. Namangan Andijan Fergana	NA	TB drugs for National DOTS Program; For Project HOPE and CDC, project manager
Red Cross		Khorezm Karakalpakstan		Food for TB patients

1,250 patients in 2000–2001. Also, 20,000 brochures and 8,000 DOTS posters were printed. This year, a new program to ensure the quality of TB drugs and appropriate drug management practices will be started in Uzbekistan with technical assistance from RPM Plus. The International Committee of the Red Cross provides food for TB patients in MSF-assisted DOTS pilot areas.

Funding

The Government reported a budget for the TB Program of about $2 million in 2003, and donor assistance of over $3 million, while annual needs would amount to about $10 million. The Government, especially the Ministry of Health, is searching for external financial aid for TB control, and it has submitted a request of $41.5 million to the Global Fund. The following needs have been identified:

- Prevalence surveys (TB disease and drug resistance).
- Communication campaign to remove stigma. Women may be more affected by stigma than men.
- Scaling up DOTS (particularly need funds for DOTS implementation in Nawoi and Jizzak Oblasts).
- Support to the national DOTS center in DOTS training.
- Publishing training materials, especially DOTS modules for GP.
- Procurement of laboratory equipment and TB drugs.
- Prisons need X-ray equipment, laboratory equipment, and TB drugs.
- Coordination of international agencies.

CHAPTER 9

CONCLUSION

The countries of Central Asia are still at the earliest stages of an HIV/AIDS epidemic. Kazakhstan, the worst affected country in Central Asia, has less than 4,000 estimated HIV cases. Until recently, the Kyrgyz Republic, Tajikistan, Turkmenistan, and Uzbekistan were scarcely affected by HIV. However, by the end of 2002, almost 6,000 HIV-infected persons were reported in these countries. The main cause for serious concern is the drug trafficking routes that pass through Central Asia. These have facilitated the growth of IV drug use in the sub region; expert estimates indicate that the region may have more than 0.5 million drug users, and outbreaks of HIV-related injecting drug use have been reported in all Central Asian countries with the exception of Turkmenistan.

The epidemic is currently concentrated among IDUs and CSWs, but it can and likely will spread to vulnerable groups such as young people, mobile populations, and sex partners of high-risk group members. However, twenty years into the epidemic, millions of young people in the sub region know little, if anything, about HIV/AIDS risks and prevention. Unprecedented numbers of young people are not completing their secondary schooling in these countries, adding to the knowledge gap. With jobs in short supply, many are at special risk of joining groups of highly vulnerable populations by resorting to injecting drug use and regular or occasional sex work.

In contrast, TB is a well-established epidemic throughout the sub region. Because of the critical nature of the MDRTB component of this epidemic, it has global significance. With pockets of MDRTB prevalence reaching more than 30 percent, the global danger of spreading resistant TB throughout ECA and beyond is of concern to all donors. TB is the most important opportunistic infection for HIV/AIDS, but for now, it is not a major overlapping epidemic concern in Central Asia. This, however, is only a matter of time before HIV infection and AIDS overlap with the epidemic of MDRTB brewing in Central Asia. In other countries affected by both epidemics, the number of TB cases has doubled and even trebled in the past decade, mainly as a result of the HIV epidemic.

There is still a window of opportunity to prevent the HIV/AIDS epidemic from exploding. National Governments must express the necessary political will and take decisive action before the epidemic of HIV expands beyond the concentrated risk groups. Young people are a priority on this front. All five countries have recognized the impending danger of an HIV epidemic, and have recently approved national programs on HIV/AIDS. Governments have taken positive steps, and have obtained grant funding to initiate the implementation of the HIV/AIDS control strategies and continue scaling up the implementation of the DOTS approach. UN agencies, the GFATM, the World Bank, USAID, the Soros Foundation/OSI, the East-West Foundation and other partner organizations have been assisting regional Governments to control the epidemics of HIV/AIDS, STIs and TB. Despite growing emphasis on a coordinated regional response, it is clear, however, that any HIV/AIDS initiative in Central Asia must deal with a cultural reluctance to confront HIV/AIDS, drug use, and sexuality.

The time to act on both HIV and TB is now, and the channels for action are multilateral and multi-sectoral. Further studies and action are necessary.

The Central Asia HIV/AIDS and TB Country Profiles were developed to inform Bank management and other stakeholders about the main characteristics of the epidemics in Central Asia; differences among the countries; and main efforts to prevent HIV/AIDS and control TB. The Country Profiles summarize the information available from regional Governments and partner organizations such as UN agencies, USAID, and the Soros Foundation/OSI.

Additional studies focusing on HIV/AIDS are being prepared for publication. These studies will contribute to identify strategies for ensuring early and effective intervention to control the epidemic at national and regional levels, considering priorities based on global evidence. The studies also aim at informing the Bank's policy dialogue and the operational work to control HIV/AIDS in Central Asia; and contributing to building up the regional partnership between Governments, civil society, UN agencies, and multilateral and bilateral agencies to prevent HIV/AIDS and STIs. Specifically, the additional studies aim to:

- Estimate the potential epidemiological and economic impact of the HIV/AIDS epidemic in Central Asia;
- Identify key stakeholders and their roles in controlling the epidemic;
- Identify gaps in strategies, policies, and legislation aimed at controlling the epidemic;
- Assess the institutional capacity, including of public health services and NGOs, to control the epidemic; and
- Prepare the Bank's communication strategy on HIV/AIDS in Central Asia.

The Bank is also carrying out the Central Asia TB Study and, in cooperation with the Government of Kazakhstan, an in-depth review of this country's TB and HIV/AIDS programs. In addition to these regional studies, the Bank has been providing technical and financial assistance to Central Asian Governments to carry out sector work and operations that tackle HIV/AIDS, STIs, and TB. The Bank's long-term investment approach is critically important to Central Asia as a part of the multi-national effort to contain these growing epidemics throughout Eastern Europe.

REFERENCES

Arndt, C. and J. Lewis. 2000. "The Macro Implications of HIV/AIDS in South Africa." Presented at IAEN conference, Durban.

Ball, A. 1998. "Policies and Interventions to Stem HIV-1 Epidemics Associated with Injecting Drug Use." *In Drug Injecting and HIV Infection: Global Dimensions and Local Responses.* London: UCL Press.

Bos, J.M., W.I. van der Meijden, W. Swart, and M.J. Postma. 2002. "Routine HIV Screening of Sexually Transmitted Disease Clinic Attendees has Favorable Cost-effectiveness Ratio in Low HIV Prevalence Settings." *AIDS* 16 (8): 1185–1187.

Burrows, D. (in preparation for publication). A Best Practice Model of Harm Reduction in the Community and in Prisons in the Russian Federation.

Busel, et al. 1998. *Prevalence of Injecting Drug Use and HIV Infection in Tashkent.* Tashkent: UNAIDS.

Carinfonet. 2000. *Health of Population and Health Care in Central Asian Republics.* WHO Information Center on Health for CAR.

Commonwealth of Australia. 2002. *Return on Investment in Needle and Syringe Programs in Australia.* Sydney: Commonwealth Department of Health and Aging.

Cox, H. and S. Hargraves. 2003. "To Treat or Not to Treat? Implementation of DOTS in Central Asia." *Lancet* 2003;361:714–716.

Cuddington, J. and Hancock. 1994. "Assessing the Impact of AIDS on the Growth Path of the Malawian Economy." *J. Dev. Econ.*, 43:363–368.

Futures Group and Instituto Nacional de Salud Publica (México). 2003 (draft). *Funding Required for the Response to HIV/AIDS in Eastern Europe and Central Asia.* Washington DC: The World Bank and UNAIDS Secretariat.

Garnett, G., et al.(unpublished manuscript). Modeling of HIV/AIDS in Russia.

Kambou G., S. Devarajan, and M. Over. 1992. "The Economic Impact of AIDS in an African Country: Simulations with a General Equilibrium Model of Cameroon." *J. African Economies*, 1:103–30.

Kokko, S. 2002. "Tuberculosis and HIV/AIDS in the Prisons of the Republic of Kyrgyzstan—Tackling the Growing Public Health Problems." Discussion Paper. Washington DC: The World Bank.

Lubin, N., A. Klaits, and I. Barsegian. 2002. *Narcotics Interdiction in Afghanistan and Central Asia: Challenges for International Assistance.* NY: The Open Society Institute. Central Eurasia Program/Network Women's Program.

MacFarlan, M. and S. Sgherri. 2001. *The Macroeconomic Impact of HIV/AIDS in Botswana.* IMF working paper WP/01/80.

Ministry of Health (Uzbekistan). 2003. Uzbekistan Health Examination Survey 2002. Preliminary Report. Tashkent.

Oostvogels, R. 2001. *Assessment of Female Sex Workers and Clients in Tashkent, Republic of Uzbekistan.* Tashkent: UNAIDS.

Oostvogels, R. and H. Mikkelsen. 1998. *Assessment of the Situation Regarding HIV and Men Who Have Sex with Men in Tashkent, Uzbekistan.* Tashkent: UNAIDS.

Regional Conference on Drug Abuse in Central Asia. *Situation Assessment and Responses.* Tashkent: UNODCCP, WHO, USAID, OSCE, Austrian Federal Ministry of Foreign Affairs and Government of Uzbekistan.

Ruhl, K., et al. 2002. "The Economic Consequences of HIV in Russia." World Bank Russia web page.

"Swiss Expert Commission Recommends Decriminalization of Drug Use." 1996. *Canadian HIV/AIDS Policy and Law Newsletter,* 2 (4).

Thomas, M. 1997. *Assessment of Commercial Sex Scene in Tashkent.* Tashkent: UNAIDS.

UNAIDS (Joint United Nations Program on HIV/AIDS). 2001. *UNAIDS-assisted Response to HIV/AIDS, STIs and Drug Abuse in Central Asian Countries.* Almaty: UNAIDS—Central Asia.

———. 2002a. *Kazakhstan Epidemiological Fact Sheet.*

———. 2002b. *Kyrgyzstan Fact Sheet.*

———. 2002c. *Report on the Global HIV/AIDS epidemic 2002.* Geneva: UNAIDS.

UNICEF. 2002. *Social Monitor: HIV/AIDS and Young People.* Florence: UNICEF.

USAID/CAR (United States Agency for International Development / Central Asia Republics). 2002. *USAID/CAR Strategy on HIV/AIDS Prevention in Central Asia 2002–2004.* Almaty: USAID Regional Mission for Central Asia.

Uzbek Association on Reproductive Health/IPPF. 2001. *UARH Work with Youth in the Field of HIV/AIDS Prevention Measures in Uzbekistan.* Tashkent: UARH

Uzbekistan Interdepartamental Working Group on HIV/AIDS. 2002. *Strategic Program on Counteraction to HIV/AIDS Epidemic Expansion in the Republic of Uzbekistan.* Tashkent: Government of Uzbekistan.

Van Het Loo, et al. 2001. *Decriminalization of Drug Use in Portugal: The Development of a Policy.* RAND Europe, Leiden, The Netherlands.

Vinokur, Godinho, Dye, and Nagelkerke. 2001. *The TB and HIV/AIDS Epidemics in the Russian Federation.* Washington: World Bank.

WHO (World Health Organization). 2001. *WHO Regional Strategy on Sexual and Reproductive Health.* Copenhagen: WHO Reproductive Health/Pregnancy Programme.

World Bank. 1997. *Confronting AIDS.* Washington D.C: the World Bank.

———. (draft under review). ESW Concept Note on Insurance, HIV/AIDS and TB Sector Work. Washington DC: The World Bank. ECSHD.

———. (draft under preparation). Project Concept Document. Washington D.C: The World Bank. ECSHD.

Zaripova, et al. 2001. *Prevalence of Injecting Drug Use and HIV-infection in the City of Samarkand.* Samarkand: MINISTRY OF HEALTH: AIDS Centre.